Nelson Yuan-sheng Kiang

rcvd 10/92

CLINICS IN DEVELOPMENTAL MEDICINE NO. 108

OTITIS MEDIA WITH EFFUSION IN CHILDREN
–The Dunedin Study

Clinics in Developmental Medicine No. 108

OTITIS MEDIA WITH EFFUSION IN CHILDREN – The Dunedin Study

DAVID CHALMERS
IAN STEWART
PHIL SILVA
ANNE MULVENA

Dunedin Multidisciplinary Health and Development Research Unit
Department of Paediatrics and Child Health
University of Otago Medical School

1989
Mac Keith Press
OXFORD: Blackwell Scientific Publications Ltd.
PHILADELPHIA: J. B. Lippincott Co.

5a Netherhall Gardens, London NW3 5RN

First published 1989

British Library Cataloguing in Publication Data

Otitis media with effusion in children.
1. Children. Middle ear. Otitis media
I. Chalmers, D. II. Series
618.92′09784

ISBN (UK) 0 632 02467 4
(USA) 0 397 48012 1

Printed in Great Britain at The Lavenham Press Ltd., Lavenham, Suffolk
Mac Keith Press is supported by **The Spastics Society, London, England**

AUTHORS' APPOINTMENTS

DAVID CHALMERS, B.A., Ph.D.	Scientific Officer, Dunedin Multidisciplinary Health and Development Research Unit, University of Otago Medical School.
IAN STEWART, M.B., Ch.B., F.R.C.S.Ed.	Head of Department of Otolaryngology/Head and Neck Surgery, University of Otago Medical School and Dunedin Hospital.
PHIL SILVA, M.A., Ph.D.	Director, Dunedin Multidisciplinary Health and Development Research Unit, University of Otago Medical School.
ANNE MULVENA, B.A., M.S.	Staff Audiologist, Audiology Department, Dunedin Hospital.

CONTENTS

FOREWORD

Otitis media and serous otitis media are very common in childhood but occur equally in the adult population. In general, the Mac Keith Press has eschewed publications about non-neurological diseases, being in the main concerned with the chronic disabling conditions of childhood and the factors which lead to them. At first sight, therefore, one might question whether the Press should be concerned with these issues. However, there has long been a suspicion that the developmental consequences of some acute illnesses may be as significant as those of many chronic neurological diseases. The exact significance of 'glue ear' in childhood is one which has increasingly concerned paediatricians, psychologists and others over the last several years.

The many studies which have been done on this problem, however, have often lacked a sound scientific base and one of the first benefits this book bestows is a comprehensive review of that literature, under a very full discussion of the methodological problems of understanding the long-term effects of otitis media with effusion (OME). Only a longitudinal study can hope to answer the question of the significance of OME: this is exactly the aim of this book.

The Dunedin Study has already been remarkable for material it has produced about the health and development of young children, and this latest monograph is a worthy addition to the many previous publications.

There are problems, of course, in particular the fact that more data relating to the ears and audiological mechanisms of the study sample were not collected at the earlier examinations. However, the very careful descriptions of the later examinations are impressive, and thus it is not surprising to find that at last some of the questions we have been asking about OME are answered by this study. What the authors demonstrate is the clear appropriateness of the publication of this volume in the *Clinics in Developmental Medicine* series, because there *are* developmental consequences of OME: 'Deficits in language development, speech articulation, reading and teacher-reported behaviour problems first identified at 5 years were found to have persisted into the mid-childhood years and were still present at age 11.' This very significant finding is clearly disturbing. As the authors comment, 'Notwithstanding the necessity for further research on both the epidemiology and developmental consequences of OME, it is evident from the findings of this and other recent studies that *there is an urgent need for the detection and management of early onset OME*' (my italics).

Unfortunately, we still know too little about the appropriate way to manage OME, but this study, giving us the basic background and natural history, emphasises the importance of that task. We can no longer say, 'He'll grow out of it—his glue ear will get better.' It clearly is vital that we pursue an active role to try to prevent the consequences that Chalmers and his co-authors describe.

MARTIN BAX

PREFACE

This monograph marks the completion of a longitudinal study of otitis media with effusion, which began in 1975. In that year, 1037 children born in Dunedin, New Zealand, three years previously, were enrolled in a longitudinal study now known as the Dunedin Multidisciplinary Health and Development Study. A history of coughs, colds, ear infections and hearing problems was obtained from the parents of each of these children during the course of a day-long series of interviews and assessments dealing with many aspects of the health and development of the sample. In 1977, the first in a series of four biennial otological and audiological assessments was conducted on the members of the sample. These assessments were made when the children were at the ages of 5, 7, 9 and 11 years. In addition to the otological and audiological assessments, the children were assessed on a wide range of health, developmental and behavioural measures as part of the larger study.

The otological and audiological assessment protocols were designed by Ian Stewart, the principal investigator for this component of the study, and administered under his supervision. Phil Silva, as Director of the Dunedin Multidisciplinary Health and Development Research Unit, had overall responsibility for the selection and administration of the various measures collected as part of the larger study. In 1984, David Chalmers, a psychologist, was employed under a Medical Research Council of New Zealand grant to analyse the otological, audiological and related data collected in the previous eight years, and to co-ordinate the writing of a comprehensive report on the study. Anne Mulvena, an audiologist, also became involved in the project at this time, as an advisor. The report was completed and presented to the Medical Research Council in December 1986. That report is presented here with some modification, including an updated literature review. Some of the material presented has appeared in previous publications by the present authors.

We are very grateful to the Medical Research Council of New Zealand for funding the study and for the generosity of the Deafness Research Foundation in providing an examining microscope. Advice and encouragement—given by Mr P. Eidsell-Moore, Chairman of the Deafness Research Foundation; Dr Bill Keith, previously Principal Audiologist with the Department of Health; Mrs Sheila Williams, Biostatistician with the Department of Preventive and Social Medicine, University of Otago Medical School; Dr Rob McGee, Deputy Director of the Dunedin Multidisciplinary Health and Development Research Unit; and Professor Graham Mortimer, Chairman of the Department of Paediatrics and Child Health, University of Otago Medical School, of which the Dunedin Multidisciplinary Health and Development Research Unit is a part—is greatly appreciated. The enormous task of collecting the data for the study was carried out very ably and efficiently by Dr Ann Simpson, Dr Sophie Narodetsky, Mrs Coralie Kirkland, and the staff of the Dunedin Multidisciplinary Health and Development Research Unit. Special thanks must go to Mrs Daphne McCallum, Ms Judith Murray-White, Ms Lynn Ross, Miss Jackie Lodge and Mrs Roslyn Sydney for typing the manuscript in its many versions, and to Mr Peter Scott for drawing the graphs. We wish to thank, also, the Editorial Board of the Mac Keith Press for their courage in stepping outside their normal brief with the publication of this volume. We are grateful for the interest, patience and attention to detail shown by the editorial staff at Mac Keith Press during the preparation of this work for publication; in particular we would like to thank Dr Martin Bax, Mr Pat Chappelle, Dr Pamela Davies and Mr Bernard Hayes. Finally, we wish to express our sincere gratitude to the children who participated in the study and to their parents, for their co-operation throughout the study.

DAVID CHALMERS
IAN STEWART
PHIL SILVA
ANNE MULVENA

1
REVIEW OF LITERATURE

Introduction

Otitis media with effusion (OME) has been identified as a significant health problem for children in the early years of life. The onset of the disease is often insidious, its course is variable, recovery may be spontaneous, and recurrence is common. The surgical procedures directed toward its treatment are held to be the most commonly performed in the 'developed' world. OME is frequently accompanied by mild hearing loss and it is widely believed that victims may suffer long-lasting developmental consequences. The validity of this belief has been the subject of debate for almost two decades.

The purpose of this report is to present the results of a longitudinal study of OME, conducted as part of a multidisciplinary investigation of the health and development of a sample of 1037 children born in Dunedin, New Zealand. The members of the cohort received comprehensive otological and audiological assessments at two-yearly intervals from 5 to 11 years of age. Various measures of psychological, educational and behavioural development were administered as part of the wider study, and perinatal histories were available to the investigators.

Definitions and classification

Classification of middle-ear effusion has been highly controversial, particularly in recent years when awareness of the importance and ubiquity of the problem has been common. Middle-ear effusion has been defined as the 'collection of fluid in the middle ear cavity' (Senturia *et al.* 1980).

The condition has at different times been labelled 'catarrhal otitis', 'serous otitis media', 'secretory otitis media', 'non-suppurative otitis media', 'mucoid ear' and, popularly, 'glue ear' (Paparella 1976, Senturia 1976, Bluestone 1984). Mawson (1976) traced the evolution of this nomenclature, noting the name-changes that have occurred as knowledge of the condition has increased. He observed that in the research literature the various terms listed above have been used 'interchangeably, and indiscriminately', leading to uncertainty over which particular manifestation of the disease is being referred to at any particular time.

At the 1979 Research Conference on Recent Advances in Otitis Media with Effusion, the *ad hoc* committee on definition and classification of otitis media advanced the term 'otitis media with effusion' (OME). It was recognized that otitis media was a 'dynamic continuing process in which the specific diagnostic term can change' (Senturia *et al.* 1980). This definition placed little emphasis on the quality of middle-ear effusion, while recognizing qualitative variations in middle-ear effusion. Acute, sub-acute and chronic effusions were all included in the term OME.

This classification was not universally accepted, particularly in Europe. There was a reluctance to accept the term 'OME' as referring to all middle-ear effusions, acute and chronic. Although it was recognized that the acute, subacute and chronic states merge into one another, it was considered that the exact chronology is not necessarily evident clinically so that precise categorization becomes difficult. On the other hand, there appeared a clear-cut clinical distinction between acutely symptomatic otitis media with pain and/or discharge, and more chronic effusions having deafness and associated developmental problems as their major clinical manifestation.

At the Third International Symposium on Recent Advances in Otitis Media with Effusion (held at Fort Lauderdale, FL, in May 1983) the apparent consensus of the previous international symposium was questioned. The consensus view of the Third International Symposium was that individual authors may use whatever nomenclature appeared appropriate, provided that it was defined (Paparella *et al.* 1985). In the light of this consensus, it is proposed to define the problem as follows.

Acute otitis media is defined as an acutely symptomatic problem, presenting with pain and/or discharge from the ear.

Otitis media with effusion (OME) is defined as a middle-ear effusion as evidenced by otomicroscopic and tympanometric findings and without the symptoms and signs of acute otitis media. No attempt is made to define the chronology of OME.

Epidemiology, natural history and risk factors

According to Klein *et al.* (1980) the benefits to be derived from epidemiological and natural history studies of otitis media (OM) are at least two-fold. On the one hand they provide an insight into the aetiology and pathogenesis of the disease and on the other they aid in the development and evaluation of intervention strategies. Several reviews of epidemiological and natural history studies have appeared during the past decade and from these much can be learned about the prevalence and incidence of OM, about factors affecting its occurrence, and about the natural course of the disease. Unfortunately, the majority of these reviews fail to differentiate between OME and other manifestations of the disease, most notably acute OM. Since the present report is concerned only with OME, the following literature review concentrates on studies directly related to this manifestation of the disease.

A brief history of research on otitis media

In a paper presented to the first international symposium on OME, Paradise (1976) observed that few studies of the epidemiology of the condition, and to his knowledge none concerned with its natural history, had been reported in the literature. At about the same time Ingram (1976), in a brief survey of the literature, noted that 'the prevalence of middle-ear disease and intermittent hearing loss is unknown'. However, he was able to identify at least two early British studies that suggested that around 17 to 19 per cent of children have at least one episode of OM, many with perforation of the tympanic membrane, before the age of 5 years. Subsequently, Brooks (1979) presented a review of studies on hearing loss in children in which he identified OME as 'the major cause of auditory dysfunction in preschool and early-grade school children'. From the results of six studies Brooks concluded that between 10 and 30 per cent of infants and preschool children are affected by OME. Furthermore, on the basis of other studies he speculated that 'not less than 90 per cent of hearing impairment and auditory system abnormality in early school age children is of the conductive type' and implied that OME played a major aetiologic role. Finally, he reviewed several studies which indicated that middle-ear disease appeared to diminish 'as a cause of hearing impairment after the age of six or seven years'.

Klein (1979) and more recently Giebink (1984) have reviewed contemporary research on factors influencing the occurrence of acute OM, including age, sex, race and socio-economic status: some reference will be made to these reviews below. Unfortunately, the only reviews of research on the natural history of OM (Howie 1975, 1979; Howie *et al.* 1976) relate to acute OM and not OME as defined for the purpose of this study.

Methodological problems

A number of criticisms have been levelled at the quality of the epidemiological and natural history studies that have appeared in the literature. These have included a failure to define the disease precisely, to distinguish between different disease types and stages, or to evaluate the validity and reliability of diagnosis, the inadequate description of populations or samples, non-random sampling, and inadequate statistical design and analysis (Klein 1979, Klein *et al.* 1980, Giebink 1984). In addition, Klein *et al.* (1980) observed that too few studies have been 'designed to yield epidemiologic information'.

Occurrence of OME

In his review of epidemiological studies prior to 1976, Paradise (1976) stated that not only were these 'disappointingly few' in number but also that they were 'difficult to compare, since some involved incidence, some point-prevalence, and some involved prevalence over time'. The incidence of a disease is described as the number of new cases that occur in a population during a specified period (Farmer and Miller 1983). The incidence rate is defined as follows.

$$\text{Incidence rate} = \frac{\text{Number of new cases of a disease in a population during a specified period}}{\text{Number of persons in the population during that period}}$$

The incidence rate, therefore, is an estimate of the risk of developing a disease during a specified period (Lilienfeld and Lilienfeld 1980).

The prevalence of a disease is described by Farmer and Miller (1983) as the number of cases in a population at a particular point in time (point prevalence) or during a specified period (period prevalence). The prevalence rate is defined as follows.

$$\text{Prevalence rate} = \frac{\text{Number of cases of a disease present in a population at a specified time or during a specified period}}{\text{Number of persons in the population at that specified time or during that specified period}}$$

Incidence and prevalence are normally expressed as rates per 1000 population (Lilienfeld and Lilienfeld 1980). In the literature on OME, however, these rates are characteristically expressed as percentages. This convention will be observed in the following review.

One popular but not particularly satisfactory method of measuring the occurrence of OME is to identify 'patient-visits' which have resulted in diagnosis of the disease. Klein (1979), for example, reported that between one-fifth and one-quarter of the children, under the age of 1 year, attending a Boston paediatric clinic were found to have OM (type unspecified). Similarly, Thompson *et al.* (1984) reported that from 3864 patient-visits made to a Tennessee health care practice by 210 children during their first two years of life, 178 cases of serous otitis media were diagnosed (4.5 per cent of visits). Finally, Reves *et al.* (1985) reported that of 264 children, aged from 3 months to 6 years, listed on the register of a general practice in north-west London, 31 per cent had evidence of middle-ear effusion on first examination. The practice served a 'deprived' population.

While such studies can provide useful information on the occurrence of OME among those children attending the practices concerned, it cannot be claimed that their findings in any way reflect the distribution of the disease in the wider population of children. The same criticism can be levelled at studies based on other very specific samples. Casselbrant *et al.* (1984, 1985), for example, reported incidence and prevalence rates for preschool children in the USA, using a sample of 103 children aged from 2 to 6 years and attending a daycare centre in a suburb of Pittsburgh, PA, over a period of two years. Incidence rates of 53 per cent and 61 per cent were reported for the first and second years of the study respectively. Prevalence rates ranged from 7 per cent in summer to 33 per cent in winter. In a second study, Casselbrant *et al.* (1986) sampled 111 children between the ages of 5 and 12 years, from a single school in suburban Pittsburgh. A cumulative incidence rate of 22 per cent per year was reported. Similarly, Okeowo (1985) reported urban and rural incidence rates for Nigerian children, based on a sample of 544 children from a single urban school and an otherwise undefined sample of 220 rural children respectively. The children were aged from 3 to 11 years. The urban rate was 4.9 per cent and the rural rate 8.2 per cent. The sampling procedures used in these studies were completely inadequate for the purpose of describing the frequency of occurrence of OME in the populations they purported to represent.

A more satisfactory standard of sampling, with wider representation and less bias, has been achieved in a number of recent studies. The majority of these have been conducted in Denmark but studies from other countries have been reported.

Lous and Fiellau-Nikolajsen (1981) studied a cohort of 387 children, all of whom started their schooling in two rural municipalities of Denmark (Hirtshals and Sindal) in 1978. In one study, Fiellau-Nikolajsen (1983*a*) screened the population of 3-year-old children in the municipality of Hjoerring, Denmark (N=456) and selected 404 of these for repeated testing over a period of one year. In a second study, Fiellau-Nikolajsen (1983*b*) examined 96 per cent of all 523 children born in the Hjoerring municipality during 1977 and 94 per cent of all 463 children born in the same municipality during the year from August 1974 to July 1975. Tos (1983) described three cohorts studied by himself and his colleagues. These included 151 children randomly selected from among those born in the Gentofte Hospital maternity ward, Copenhagen, between January and April, 1977 (Poulsen and Tos 1978, Tos *et al.* 1979*b*), all children born during the first 10 days of every month in 1975 in two municipalities of Copenhagen County (Tos *et al.* 1978, 1983*b*), and all children born during the first 10 days of every month in 1976 in the same two municipalities (Tos 1983). Birch and Elbrond (1986) sampled 319 children, aged 1 to 6 years, from a population of 709 children in home or private day care in a small municipality (population 17,000) of Denmark.

Van Cauwenberge and Kluyskens (1984) examined 2069 children attending different Belgian kindergartens during the period May 1979 to January 1980. In a Canadian study reported by Lamothe *et al.* (1981), 958 of the 1127 children attending the first grade of all elementary schools in the Sherbrooke metropolitan area were examined for OME. Holmquist *et al.* (1987) examined 817 children from eight primary schools distributed among four educational districts in Kuwait. Finally, Rach *et al.* (1986) recruited a cohort of 1439 children born in the city of Nijmegen in the Netherlands. Of these, 87 per cent received impedance testing at the age of 2 years. Incidence and prevalence rates taken from these studies are presented in the following two sections.

INCIDENCE OF OME IN CHILDREN

Relatively few of the above studies reported incidence rates for OME in children. Lous and Fiellau-Nikolajsen (1981) reported a rate of 25 per cent per year for the 7-year-olds in their study. Fiellau-Nikolajsen (1983*a*) identified 88 new cases of OME in a sample of 404 3-year-olds, examined on four occasions over a six-month period, giving an incidence rate of approximately 22 per cent for that period. Fiellau-Nikolajsen acknowledged that such an estimate is not necessarily accurate, given that no account is taken of cases which appear and subside between examinations. Finally, a mean incidence rate of 27 per cent per month for children aged from 1 to 7 years, in home or private day care, was reported by Birch and Elbrond (1986). The rates were fairly consistent across age-groups. Although expressed in different time periods, the findings of these three Danish studies suggest that the incidence of OME during the first seven years of life is in the vicinity of 25 per cent per year. This estimate is somewhat lower than the 53 to 61 per cent reported by Casselbrant *et al.* (1984, 1985) for children in Pittsburgh, PA. A final estimate of incidence is provided by Tos (1983), who suggested that almost 80 per cent of children will have at least one episode of OME during the first seven years of life.

With regard to the incidence of OME in New Zealand, the NZ Board of Health Committee on Hearing (1984) reported that no reliable rates were available for preschool children. From limited historical data made available by the Christchurch Child Development Study, however, they reported that 'approximately 25 per cent of children have episodes of otitis media in any one year between birth and age five'. This estimate is consistent with those of the Danish studies reviewed above. It is unfortunate, however, that the Christchurch data were based on patient-visits to general practitioners and that the types of OM involved were not specified.

TABLE 1.1
Summary of studies reporting prevalence of otitis media with effusion

Authors	*Location*	*Age of children*	*Season*	*Children N*	*Ears N*	*Identification criterion*	*Prevalence**
Poulsen and Tos (1978)	Denmark	2–4 days	Winter	150	300	B tympanogram†	0.0
		3 mths	Spring		252	,,	0.0
		6 mths	Summer		238	,,	1.3
Tos *et al.* (1979*b*)	,,	9 mths	Autumn		236	,,	4.0
		1 year	Winter		206	,,	13.0
Tos (1983)	,,	15 mths	Spring		132	,,	14.0
		18 mths	Summer		132	,,	12.0
		21 mths	Autumn		132	,,	19.0
		2 yrs	Winter		132	,,	14.0
		,,	,,		508	,,	14.0
		,,	Spring		480	,,	11.0
		,,	Summer		440	,,	7.0
Tos *et al.* (1978)	,,	,,	Autumn	278	556	,,	11.0
Rach *et al.* (1986)	Netherlands	,,	,,	1099		,,	26.0
		,,	Winter			,,	39.0
		,,	Spring			,,	32.0
		,,	Summer			,,	24.0
Fiellau-Nikolajsen (1983*a*)	Denmark	3 yrs	,,	404	808	,,	13.7
		,,	Autumn		808	,,	13.7
		,,	,,		808	,,	13.0
		,,	Winter		808	,,	16.0
Fiellau-Nikolajsen (1983*b*)	,,	,,	,,	504	1001	,,	9.8
		,,	Summer	435	867	,,	8.2
		,,	Autumn	420	840	,,	9.3
		,,	,,	411	822	,,	8.8
		,,	Winter	404	808	,,	10.0

Tos (1983)	„	„	„	150	132	„	11.0
		„	„	278	404	„	11.0
		4 yrs	„	150	132	„	18.0
		„	„	278	368	„	14.0
		„	„	373	746	„	14.0
		„	Spring		670	„	11.0
		„	Summer		666	„	10.0
		„	Autumn		576	„	14.0
		5 yrs	Winter	278	280	„	11.0
Tos *et al.* (1983*b*)	„	„	„	360	628	„	18.0
Fiellau-Nikolajsen (1983*b*)	„	6 yrs	„	498	986	„	6.1
Tos *et al.* (1983*b*)	„	„	„	360	538	„	14.0
		7 yrs	„		590	„	7.0
Lous and Fiellau-Nikolajsen (1981)	„	„	Summer	384		„	5.7**
		„	Autumn	382		„	9.0**
		„	Summer	374		„	2.4**
Van Cauwenberge and Kluyskens (1984)	Belgium	2–6 yrs	—	2069	3898	Flat tympanogram; absent stapedial reflex; otoscopic examination	12.0
Lamothe *et al.* (1981)	Canada	6–8 yrs	—	958		Otoscopic examination	7.0**
Holmquist *et al.* (1987)	Kuwait	7–9 yrs	Winter	817	1634	B tympanogram	12.2
			Spring				9.5

*Prevalence per 100 *ears* except where noted. **Prevalence per 100 *children*.
†Flat curve and impedance slope <0.1 (Jerger 1970).

PREVALENCE OF OME IN CHILDREN

A greater proportion of the studies identified in the foregoing section reported prevalence rates for OME in children. Point prevalence rates for each of these studies are presented in the first section of Table 1.1.

Because the prevalence of OME varies with age, the rates shown in Table 1.1 are listed according to age. The season during which the prevalence was assessed has been identified, as this is another factor which has been shown to influence the occurrence of the disease. Three studies which each provided a single prevalence rate for children varying in age (Lamothe *et al.* 1981, Van Cauwenberge and Kluyskens 1984, Holmquist *et al.* 1987) have been included at the foot of Table 1.1 because they provide prevalence rates for a further three countries—Belgium, Canada and Kuwait.

It will be noted that for the studies listed in the first section of the table, a type B tympanogram* was taken as evidence of OME. Tos *et al.* (1983*b*) included ears with open grommets as type B cases in their study of OME in preschool schildren. Fiellau-Nikolajsen (1983*a*), on the other hand, specifically excluded children with grommets from the analysis of prevalence data. Of the studies reported at the foot of the table, Holmquist *et al.* (1987) based their prevalence rates on tympanogram type alone, Lamothe *et al.* (1981) used evidence from otoscopy alone, and Van Cauwenberge and Kluyskens (1984) used both impedance audiometry and otoscopy to identify cases.

It is evident from the studies listed in Table 1.1 that the prevalence of OME varies about a median rate of approximately 13 per cent between the ages of 1 and 6 years. The only evidence available for children younger than 1 year indicates that the prevalence of OME increases from 1.3 per cent at 6 months to 4.0 per cent at 9 months, reaching 13.0 per cent at 12 months (Poulsen and Tos 1978, Tos *et al.* 1979*b*). The evidence from one Danish study (Tos 1983, Tos *et al.* 1983*b*) suggests that at the age of 7 years, the prevalence rate drops sharply to about 7 per cent, while that of another Danish study (Lous and Fiellau-Nikolajsen 1981), conducted over a period of 12 months, indicates that this decline continues with increasing age. When tested at the beginning of that study, 5.7 per cent of the 7-year-olds had type B tympanograms; 12 months later the rate had declined to 2.4 per cent.

The above figures are supported by the evidence of Van Cauwenberge and Kluyskens (1984), who reported that the prevalence of OME in Belgian children ranging in age from 2½ to 6 years was 12 per cent, and by that of Lamothe *et al.* (1981) who reported that for Canadian children aged from 6 to 8 years the prevalence rate was 7 per cent. At variance, however, are the rates of 12.2 per cent (winter) and 9.5 per cent (spring) reported by Holmquist *et al.* (1987), from their study of Kuwaiti children aged between 7 and 9½ years.

It is clear that there is considerable variation in the prevalence rates reported, both within and between studies. For children aged from 1 to 6 years the rates range from 6.1 per cent (Fiellau-Nikolajsen 1983*b*) to 39 per cent (Rach *et al.* 1986). Some of the variation may be attributed to seasonal fluctuations, but there is also evidence of differences between researchers and/or locations. For example,

*For a definition of tympanogram types, see p. 18.

while Fiellau-Nikolajsen (1983*b*) reported an average prevalence of 9.2 per cent among 3-year olds, Tos (1983) reported an average of 11 per cent for the same age-group. A dramatic variation between countries is evident in the rates reported for 2-year-olds. Rach *et al.* (1986) reported seasonal rates for the Netherlands ranging from 24 to 39 per cent, while those reported by Tos (1983) for Denmark ranged from 7 to 14 per cent. Apart from a very cold winter and wet summer during the data collection period, Rach *et al.* (1986) could offer no plausible explanation for the very high rates recorded for their cohort.

Turning now to evidence of the prevalence of OME in New Zealand children, there is little useful information to be found in the literature in this regard. The same criticisms regarding methods of research and the reporting of results that have been levelled at the international literature can be applied to the New Zealand literature also. A review of research on ear infection by Clements and Joseph (1981) identified a small number of studies which had reported prevalence rates for OME. The same studies were referred to in the recently published report of the New Zealand Board of Health Committee on Hearing (1984). In both of these reviews a number of studies were referred to in which prevalence rates for OM were reported but the specific type or types of OM concerned were not specified.

Clements and Joseph described the results of a study reported by Asher and Short (1978) in which 300 (predominantly Maori) children aged from 1 month to 15 years were examined for ear infection. Of these, 0.7 per cent were reported to have 'serous otitis media' and a further 9.3 per cent were found to have retracted tympanic membranes, a sign of middle-ear effusion. In another study of 277 (again, predominantly Maori) school- and preschool children, Hamilton *et al.* (1980) found on microscopic examination that 14.4 per cent had OME. Separate age-group rates for these children were reported but, because it is not clear how these were calculated, little reliance can be placed on them. That study was conducted in November, during the New Zealand spring season. Finally, in a study of hearing screening methods in nine South Auckland primary schools, Maynard and Keith (1981) found that of 533 new school entrants, 8 per cent failed an impedance screen in their better ear (as determined by a pure-tone screen) and 17 per cent failed in their worse ear. The criterion for failure was a type B tympanogram or a type B/C tympanogram (intermediate between types B and C) in the absence of an acoustic reflex. Combining the results for both ears gives an overall failure rate of 12 per cent for the sample. Although not intended as prevalence rates for OME, these results provide a further estimate of the occurrence of this disorder in New Zealand children. Maynard and Keith's (1981) study was conducted during September and October, in the New Zealand spring season.

The rates reported in the above studies suggest that the prevalence of OME in New Zealand children is similar to that in children of other countries. Given the small number of studies reviewed, the wide range of ages considered in two of the studies, the poorly defined terminology in one study, the lack of representativeness in sampling, and the other methodological problems mentioned above, these rates can be taken only as very tentative estimates of the prevalence of OME in New Zealand children.

Natural history

Recent studies have considered three aspects of the natural history of OME: duration, recurrence and spontaneous improvement. The evidence relating to each of these aspects is described below.

DURATION

In a review of natural history studies, Giebink (1984) described two longitudinal studies in which the duration of OME had been traced. These studies found that following a first acute episode of OME, over 50 per cent of sufferers still had the disease after two weeks, over 20 per cent after four weeks, 15 per cent after six weeks, 10 per cent after 12 weeks, and for 6 per cent it was still present after 16 weeks. Lous and Fiellau-Nikolajsen (1981) reported that for 100 6-year-olds with OME the average duration of the disease was 1.8 months. Over half of these children (56 per cent) recovered within one month while 16 per cent had the disease for six months or longer. Episodes of OME commencing in the winter months were found to persist longer than those commencing in the summer. In a study of 404 3-year-olds, Fiellau-Nikolajsen (1983*a*) found that of 78 children with OME at the first of four examinations made over a six-month period, 36 per cent had it for less than four weeks, 23 per cent had it for up to 12 weeks, and a further 9 per cent recovered within 24 weeks. For 32 per cent of the children the disease persisted for over 24 weeks.

From the investigation of three cohorts of children ranging in age from birth to 7 years, Tos (1983) found that OME, as evidenced by a type B tympanogram, persisted most frequently for between three and six months. Since the period between examinations was never less than three months, no indication was given of the exact duration of those episodes resolving within three months. In the first cohort, OME was found to persist for one to two years in 7.6 per cent of ears; in the second, in 2.3 per cent of ears; and in the third, in 3.1 per cent. Tos *et al.* (1984) examined the duration of OME in these three cohorts, and on the basis that 80 per cent of preschool children had at least one episode of OME before school age, drew the following preliminary conclusions.

1. Single episodes of one to six months duration occurred in 15 per cent of ears.
2. Short but recurring episodes of one to six months duration occurred in about 25 per cent of ears.
3. Protracted episodes of six to 12 months duration occurred in 15 per cent of ears.
4. Protracted cases that improved but deteriorated again had an incidence of about 15 per cent.
5. Very protracted cases of one to four years duration had an incidence of 10 per cent.

Lamothe *et al.* (1981) reported a study in which 64 children, ranging in age from 6 to 8 years and who had been found to have OME at one examination, were given further examinations after three and six weeks. After three weeks 40 still had OME, and for 19 of these the condition persisted after six weeks. Of the 24 children for whom the condition had normalized within three weeks, nine had OME again at the six week examination.

Casselbrant *et al.* (1984) examined 64 children, aged 2 to 5 years, at monthly intervals over a period of one year. 34 (52 per cent) developed OME at least unilaterally during this period. Of these, 60 per cent resolved within one month and a further 20 per cent within two months. Confirmation of this finding was obtained by Casselbrant *et al.* (1985) in a second year of observations made on the same sample.

Finally, in 79 children whose surgery for the treatment of persistent OME was delayed for two-and-a-half years, the disease was found to have persisted in 69 per cent of ears (Leiberman and Bartal 1986). The authors reported that the ages of these children ranged from 2 to 12 years but failed to indicate if there was any relationship between age and spontaneous resolution of the OME.

In summary, while there is wide variation between studies, the available data suggest that most cases of OME are of short duration, with most (36 to 77 per cent) resolving in less than one month. Similarly, reports of the numbers of chronic cases vary widely, with durations of 12 weeks or more having been reported in from 9.5 to 32 per cent of children with OME. Protracted OME, lasting from one to four years, has been found in from 2.3 to 10 per cent of cases.

RECURRENCE

Lous and Fiellau-Nikolajsen (1981) found that of 87 7-year-olds with OME, 54 had only one episode, 29 had two episodes, and four had three episodes during a 12 month period. Tos (1983) reported that among the cohorts he and his colleagues had studied, approximately 40 per cent of children had recurring episodes of OME. Casselbrant *et al.* (1984, 1985) reported recurrent episodes of OME in 33 per cent of ears followed over a two year period. From a review of five studies, Giebink (1984) concluded that the timing and number of previous episodes of OME have an influence on the course of the disease. That is, the risk of *recurrent* episodes of OME is increased with each successive episode, particularly if the first of these occurs during the first year of life. Giebink (1984) further concluded that the risk of *persistent* OME is greater among children under 2 years of age.

The New Zealand Board of Health Committee on Hearing (1984) examined data for a group of children followed for their first five years of life by the Christchurch Child Development Study. As noted earlier, these data were based on visits to the general practitioner for OM and included all types of OM. Between 10 and 13 per cent of these children were found to have had OM in consecutive years; 18 per cent had had OM in at least three of their first five years of life.

SPONTANEOUS IMPROVEMENT

Natural history studies involving repeated tympanometric testing have demonstrated the transient nature of middle-ear pressure. Lous and Fiellau-Nikolajsen (1981) obtained tympanograms at monthly intervals from 345 7-year-olds during the course of a single year. The middle-ear status of 70 per cent of the children changed one or more times during the course of the study; for 17 per cent it changed five or more times; and for 25 per cent it differed on all occasions tested. Only 30 per cent of the children in that study had type A tympanograms, or normal ears, at all tests. Of the 100 children who had OME, 90 per cent improved to a type C or type A tympanogram during the 12 months of the study, with 76 per cent recovering completely. A similar pattern of change in middle-ear status over repeated tympanometric tests was reported by Tos (1983). In all three cohorts investigated by Tos and his associates, over half of the ears tested changed tympanogram type during the period in which they were being observed. Tos (1983) reported that for the first year of life the rate of spontaneous improvement from type B to type A or C tympanograms was 25 per cent. During the second, third and fourth years of life, the rate of spontaneous improvement from a type B tympanogram was more than 50 per cent. Spontaneous improvement was greatest during the summer months (76 per cent) and least during the winter months (19 to 27 per cent). In reference to an earlier study (Tos 1980), he cautioned that spontaneous improvement of type B does not necessarily imply normalization of the condition and that frequently type B improves to type C_2 (middle-ear pressure more negative than –200mmH_2O) which may persist for a long period and may then deteriorate to type B again. Renvall *et al.* (1982) obtained tympanograms from a group of 4-year-old children who had failed a pure-tone screening test (>20dB HTL in the frequency range 125 to 8000Hz). Of 144 ears with either a flat tympanogram (N=40) or with middle-ear pressure between –150 and –400mmH_2O (N=104), 39 per cent had normalized after six weeks and a further 21 per cent after 12 weeks. Finally, in a study in which daily tympanograms were obtained from 57 children over a period of four weeks, Birch and Elbrond (1985) found that the status of 61 per cent of ears changed during this time. In 72 per cent of cases with type B tympanograms, these persisted for less than two weeks.

In one of two New Zealand studies, Hamilton *et al.* (1980) re-assessed 163 children four months after an initial assessment. Of these, 65 per cent had improved from a type B tympanogram to either a type A or a type C tympanogram, 9 per cent had deteriorated from type A or type C to type B, and 26 per cent had remained the same. Of the 30 children who were found to have OME at the first assessment, 20 had resolved, two had perforations and eight were unchanged. In the other study, Maynard and Keith (1981) conducted impedance audiometry on 282 new school entrants who six weeks earlier had failed either a pure-tone or impedance screening test. Of these children, 10 per cent had improved when tested again, 6 per cent had deteriorated, and 83 per cent recorded the same result as before. Of the 89 children who failed the impedance audiometry, 33 per cent had normal tympanograms after six weeks.

Risk factors

An important emphasis of recent research has been toward identification of those factors which influence the occurrence of otitis media. Klein (1979) and Klein *et al.* (1980) categorized these factors into *host* (sex, age, race, social, cultural, hygiene, nutrition, family history, immunologic, physiologic and pathologic differences), *environmental* (climate, season, housing, crowding and situation), and *aetiologic* (micro-organisms, toxic substances and antigens). Since the present report is concerned with only the first two groups, recent findings relating to these are reviewed below. Reviews by Klein (1979) and Giebink (1984) are referred to. Only those studies not examined by either of these authors are described directly here. While the reviews by Klein and Giebink frequently combine the findings of studies on different manifestations of OM, the present survey of literature is restricted largely to those which address OME directly.

HOST FACTORS

Age. Klein (1979) and Giebink (1984) noted that OM, in general, has been found to occur most frequently among infants and young children. It is most prevalent in children under 7 years of age and its incidence is greatest during the first two years of life. This general picture for OM was shown also to be true for OME, when findings on the prevalence and incidence of the condition were reviewed above. Evidence from a number of studies has indicated that the prevalence of OME rises to a plateau of around 13 per cent at 1 year, continuing until the age of 6, after which it declines steadily. Fiellau-Nikolajsen (1983*b*) compared point prevalence rates for the same children at 3 years (9.8 per cent) and 6 years (6.1 per cent), finding a significant improvement in middle-ear status over this period. He concluded, however, that the annual improvement in middle-ear status during this time 'could only be very slight'. Casselbrant *et al.* (1984) reported a reduction in the incidence of OME from 69 to 25 per cent between the ages of 2 and 5 years.

Sex. The evidence on sex differences presented by Klein (1979) and Giebink (1984) is equivocal, with some studies indicating a greater frequency of OM among males (61 to 70 per cent of cases) and others reporting no significant sex difference. Similarly, there is some evidence that OME occurs more frequently in males (59 to 72 per cent of cases) than in females. Poulsen and Tos (1978) examined the middle-ear pressure of infants at birth, 3 months and 6 months, and found significant differences between males and females. Fiellau-Nikolajsen (1983*b*) found no significant difference between boys and girls in the prevalence of OME, but reported a significant difference between the sexes in the duration of the condition. In that study, 40 per cent of girls normalized after one month compared with only 6 per cent of boys. A similar pattern was reported by Lamothe *et al.* (1981) who found that after six weeks, resolution of OME had occurred in 51 per cent of girls compared with 20.7 per cent of boys. They reported, however, that the difference was not statistically significant. Tos and Poulsen (1979), in their study of 2-year olds, found that significantly more boys than girls had type B tympanograms during the summer months. Finally, Casselbrant *et al.* (1984) found that significantly more boys (64 per cent) than girls (37 per cent) developed OME during the course of a year-long study in which monthly examinations were conducted.

Race. Klein (1979) and Giebink (1984) noted that the results of several North American studies have indicated that the incidence of OM is higher among the Eskimo, American Indian and Hispanic populations than among North American Caucasians. Black children, however, appeared to have a lower incidence of OM than Caucasian children and this has been attributed to anatomical differences in the bony Eustachian tube. In one recent investigation of OME which has considered this factor, Thompson *et al.* (1984) found that in a sample of 210 children under 2 years of age, the incidence of OME in Caucasian children was over twice that of Black children.

In a recently reported survey of ear disease in Australian Aborigines, Sunderman and Dyer (1984) examined 3165 children—73 per cent of the child population of the Kimberley region of Australia. Approximately equal numbers of Aboriginal, non-Aboriginal and mixed-blood children were examined. Sunderman and Dyer found that 42 per cent of the Aboriginal and mixed-blood children had OME, characterized by a type B tympanogram, significant hearing loss and, at myringotomy, middle-ear effusion, as compared to only 21 per cent of the non-Aboriginal children.

The literature on acute OM in New Zealand children provides conflicting evidence regarding the effect of race on prevalence. Hood and Elliott (1975) reported a significantly higher prevalence of illness, with earache or discharging ear as one sympton, in Caucasian children than in Maori children. Stanhope *et al.* (1978), on the other hand, reported a significantly higher prevalence of perforated and scarred tympanic membranes in Maori children than in Caucasian children. In a study of 492 Tokelauan children under the age of 5 years, whose families had migrated to New Zealand, 21 per cent were found to have OM (Tonkin 1977). No comparative figures were provided in the report of this study.

Lines (1977) reported that of 453 pupils of an Auckland secondary school who were given a 'fuull clinical examination', 117 were found to have 'ear disease' including OME, scarring or perforation of the drums. Children of four racial groups were examined and Lines reported prevalence rates for 'ear disease' of 22.6 per cent for European children, 22.7 per cent for Maori children, 26.5 per cent for Asian children and 33.1 per cent for Pacific Island Polynesian children. Lines further reported, however, that of 632 pupils at the school who underwent pure-tone and impedance audiometry, only 44 were 'referred for further evaluation'. Of these, 26 were diagnosed by the audiologist to have eustachian tube obstruction and/or OME. It appears, therefore, that the overall prevalence of OME amongst the pupils was less than 4 per cent.

Finally, in a study of hearing screening methods, Greville (1977) found that significantly more Polynesian and Asian secondary school children failed pure-tone and impedance audiometry than did Caucasian children attending the same school. Maori children, however, did not differ significantly from the other racial groups in this sample and in a second study involving 6-year old Maori and Caucasian children there was, again, no difference between the failure rates of the two groups.

There seems to be evidence, therefore, that there are racial differences in the prevalence of OM in general and OME in particular. For New Zealand, however, the existing evidence is limited and contradictory.

Other host factors. Van Cauwenberge and Kluyskens (1984) found that 'very low birthweight' (defined as 'under 2.4kg'), small skull circumference and short birth length were significant risk factors in OME. Black (1985) investigated a variety of perinatal factors, including type and place of delivery, gestation, birthweight and admission to a special baby-care unit and found no evidence that any were associated with the occurrence of OME. Neither did he find any evidence of an association between OME and a variety of antenatal events, including raised blood pressure, anaemia, antepartum haemorrhage, influenza and rubella. Likewise he was unable to find evidence of a relationship between OME and exposure to scans, drugs, X-rays or amniocentesis during pregnancy.

It has been suggested that persistent amniotic fluid in the middle-ear may be related to middle-ear effusions in later infancy (Jaffe 1980). Amniotic debris, with an associated inflammatory reaction, has been demonstrated in the middle ears of neonates dying from other causes (DeSa 1973, 1977, 1983).

Poulsen and Tos (1978) and Tos *et al.* (1978) found no significant differences between left and right ears in the prevalence of OME but Lamothe *et al.* (1981) reported a significantly greater resolution of OME in right (56.7 per cent) than in left (18.4 per cent) ears over three- and six-week examination periods.

ENVIRONMENTAL FACTORS

Season. Evidence of seasonal variations in the prevalence of otitis media is well established, with the highest occurrence being in the winter months and the lowest in the summer months (Klein 1979, Giebink 1984). These variations have been related to seasonal changes in the prevalence of upper respiratory infection. This pattern of seasonal variation has been confirmed in a number of recent studies of OME (Tos and Poulsen 1979; Fiellau-Nikolajsen 1979, 1983*b*; Lous and Fiellau-Nikolajsen 1981; Van Cauwenberge and Kluyskens 1984; Casselbrant *et al.* 1984, 1985; Rach *et al.* 1986; Holmquist *et al.* 1987).

Smoking. There is some evidence that the presence of cigarette smokers in a child's household increases the risk of persistent OME (Giebink 1984). Households with more than one adult cigarette smoker were found by Kraemer *et al.* (1984) to significantly increase the risk of chronic middle-ear effusions. Neither Van Cauwenberge and Kluyskens (1984) nor Black (1985) found strong evidence of such a relationship, although the latter found a slightly higher proportion of cases than controls had been exposed to cigarette smoking. Van Cauwenberge and Kluyskens (1984), however, reported that if a mother smoked more than 15 cigarettes each day during pregnancy her child had a higher risk of OME than if she were a non-smoker.

Exposure in group day-care. Studies reviewed by Giebink (1984) indicated that group day-care increases the risk of acute OM. The same has been found to be true for OME. Tos and Poulsen (1979) reported a higher prevalence of type B tympanograms, during summer, for children attending public day nurseries (14.0 per cent) than for those in home or private day nurseries (4.5 per cent). Fiellau-Nikolajsen (1983*b*) found that the duration of OME was longer for 3-year-olds in day-care centres than for those in home care. In a case–control study, Black (1985) found that cases attended day-care centres more often than had controls. Kraemer *et al.* (1984), however, found no association between chronic middle-ear effusions and exposure to other children.

Epidemiology, natural history, and risk factors: conclusions

It is evident from the literature reviewed above that there are significant deficiencies in existing knowledge regarding the epidemiology, natural history, and aetiology of OME. The conclusions drawn above regarding the occurrence of the disease relied heavily on studies conducted in the northern hemisphere and particularly in Denmark. Comparatively little is known regarding these aspects of OME in New Zealand.

Although it is recognized clinically that the occurrence of OME begins to decline at about 6 or 7 years of age, none of the studies reviewed above monitored the occurrence of the disease beyond that age. One of the purposes of the Dunedin study was to determine the prevalence of the disease in children aged between 9 and 11 years. A similar paucity of epidemiological data was available for children under 3 years of age. This is a serious gap in present knowledge, particularly in view of the evidence, to be described later, of an association between OME and language delay in preschool children.

The few studies which have reported incidence rates suggest that the risk of children developing OME at least once during their first five or six years of life is very high. Further confirmation of the level of risk is needed, especially in New Zealand where only limited data on the incidence of OME were available.

Wide variations in the duration of the disease have been reported. This can be attributed partly to the design of these studies. For instance, by examining children at three-monthly intervals Tos (1983) was unable to identify episodes of shorter duration and thus was unable to confirm the findings of other researchers who had reported that most episodes of OME resolve within one month.

The survey of research concerned with risk factors indicated that for many of these factors (*e.g.* sex, socio-economic status, nutrition and allergy) the evidence was equivocal, and further research was required.

The quality of research on OME continues to be a problem, with a lack of sophistication in design and analysis limiting its value.

Identification and diagnosis

Until recently, a lack of awareness of OME and a failure to appreciate its possible consequences, together with inefficient methods of detection, have combined to exacerbate the difficulties inherent in studying the disease. The nature of the identification and diagnostic procedures involved in the detection of OME varies according to the situation, be it a community, clinical or research setting.

While OME is frequently associated with hearing loss, it is just as likely to be asymptomatic. It may arise insidiously and painlessly, it may produce only low grade discomfort, or it may be the result of an incompletely resolved acute otitis media (Stewart 1980). The course of the disease is variable and it may resolve spontaneously. The efficiency of any one test to identify the conditon is dependent on its ability to take those factors into account. Currently, identification of OME is based on the results of five main methods of detection. These are listed below and discussed in subsequent sections.

1. History: retrospective gathering of information from the child or parents (frequently unreliable unless backed up by accompanying medical evidence or reports).
2. Otoscopy (including microscopy): examination of the ears by an experienced clinician to determine the presence or absence of outer and middle-ear pathology.

3. Impedance audiometry (acoustic immittance): an objective measure of mobility and compliance of the tympanic membrane, pressure of the middle-ear cavity, and presence or absence of middle-ear muscle reflexes to auditory stimuli. Although 'acoustic immittance' is slowly replacing 'impedance audiometry' as the favoured term for this measure, it is not yet generally accepted by audiologists. For this reason the latter term has been used in this report.
4. Pure-tone audiometry: obtaining pure-tone air and bone conduction thresholds to measure the degree of hearing loss which may be attributable to the presence of OME.
5. Tympanocentesis/myringotomy: surgical investigation of the middle-ear contents (also permits microbiological/biochemical studies). This method of detection was not used in the present study and so will not be described further here.

History

While it is important to obtain a history of the child's general development, the degree to which parents can accurately relate the incidence of symptoms pertinent to OME varies, particularly as the disease is asymptomatic in many children. Therefore, more attention is focused here on the remaining detection methods.

Otoscopy

Use of the otoscope, including the pneumatic otoscope, enables the clinician to examine the tympanic membrane and to classify it according to whether OME or its sequelae are present or absent. The pneumatic otoscope requires that an airtight seal be obtained in the external auditory meatus and further judgements can be made regarding the mobility of the tympanic membrane by alternating positive and negative pressure in the external auditory meatus.

Use of the examining microscope has permitted a more detailed evaluation of the tympanic membrane, although availability is restricted to well equipped facilities with clinicians experienced in its use. Pneumatic otoscopy may also be used in conjunction with the examining microscope.

Excluding invasive surgical techniques, micro-otoscopy is generally accepted as the reference against which other tests are validated. The highest standard of otoscopy is achieved with an experienced clinician employing microscope and pneumatic otoscope.

Few studies prior to 1979 considered the validity of otoscopic findings or made any attempt to ensure that inter- and intra-observer reliability was of an acceptable standard (Bluestone and Cantekin 1979). Jordan (1972) reported only 60 per cent inter-observer agreement in 20 ears, regarding the normality versus abnormality of the tympanic membrane. In contrast, Stewart *et al.* (1983) reported greater than 99 per cent agreement between two examiners in 468 ears.

In investigations of the disease it is important to classify the state of the tympanic membrane into distinct categories, in order to enable detailed analyses to take place. Bluestone and Cantekin (1979) outlined the variables involved in otoscopic examination, under five general headings: (1) external canal condition; (2) appearance of tympanic membrane; (3) position of tympanic membrane; (4)

mobility of tympanic membrane; (5) other abnormalities of tympanic membrane and middle ear.

Because of the dynamic nature of the condition, correlation of all test results requires that they be carried out as near to simultaneously as possible, ideally within the space of a few minutes. As each method of identification does not measure exactly the same variable, perfect correlations are not possible (Brooks 1979). For example, myringotomy gives no indication of middle-ear pressure. Similarly, while the degree of conductive loss may give an indication of the amount of fluid in the middle-ear cavity, myringotomy is required to check the viscosity of the fluid (Bluestone *et al.* 1973).

Impedance audiometry

Impedance audiometry, in contrast to pure-tone audiometry, is a test especially designed to evaluate the integrity of the middle-ear system. Three measures are typically included and are as follows.

1. Tympanometry, which is the measurement of the compliance changes of the tympanic membrane as air pressure is varied in the external canal (Northern and Grimes 1978).
2. Static compliance, which is a measure of the compliance of the tympanic membrane and the middle-ear system.
3. Acoustic or stapedial muscle reflex thresholds, which assess the integrity of the reflex neural pathways and provide further information regarding the middle ear.

Impedance audiometry requires little co-operation from the patient once an airtight seal has been obtained in the external auditory meatus. It is objective and has been found to have high degrees of sensitivity and specificity in the identification of OME (Haughton 1977, Orchik *et al.* 1978, Fiellau-Nikolajsen 1980). Several comparatively recent studies have examined the predictive value of impedance audiometry, with varied results. In a longitudinal study of children in the first two years of life Wright *et al.* (1985) found impedance audiometry to be high in specificity (86 per cent) but low in sensitivity (58 per cent) when tested against pneumatic otoscopy. Marchant *et al.* (1986) reported high sensitivity (94 per cent) when tested against tympanocentesis and Gates *et al.* (1986) found fluid present at myringotomy in 83 per cent of subjects identified by impedance audiometry to be at high risk of effusion.

Tympanometric patterns have been classified in various ways but typically are divided into one of three major categories (Jerger 1970, Renvall *et al.* 1980):

Type A: normal middle-ear pressure ($\pm 100mmH_2O$) and normal compliance (0.3 to $1.5cm^3$).

Type B: flat or rounded tympanogram with no distinct pressure peak and low compliance ($<0.3cm^3$).

Type C: middle-ear pressure more negative than $-100mmH_2O$.

These patterns provide much of the information required to assess middle-ear function or status. The type C tympanogram is frequently associated with OM either in its initial stages or when resolving, while the type B tympanogram generally typifies the presence of OME (Fiellau-Nikolajsen 1980).

When the middle-ear system is stimulated by a sound of sufficiently high intensity, the stapedius muscle contracts reflexively, thereby increasing the tension of the tympanic membrane and reducing the compliance of the middle-ear system. This acoustic reflex is usually elicited at between 70 and 100dB above the pure-tone threshold. If a conductive hearing loss is present, the stimulus has to overcome the degree of loss before the reflex will be elicited. When conductive pathology is present, the stapedius reflex is usually absent either because of ossicular chain pathology or because the tiny change in compliance caused by stapedius contraction is undetectable against a major compliance change. Absence of the stapedius reflex has been advanced as an aid to detection of OME but its value is disputed.

ALTERNATIVES TO IMPEDANCE AUDIOMETRY

The acoustic otoscope, a recently developed instrument, is a commercially available alternative to impedance audiometry and has the advantage that measures do not require an airtight seal in the outer ear canal, are less affected by cerumen, and require only minimal passive co-operation. The operational principle is similar to impedance audiometry, involving partial cancellation of incident sound by sound reflected back from the tympanic membrane (Teele and Teele 1984). Although both high sensitivity (correct detection of those with fluid) and high specificity (correct rejection of those without fluid) have been achieved with the acoustic otoscope in a number of studies (Teele and Teele 1984, Schwartz and Schwartz 1987, Oyiborhoro *et al.* 1987), one comparatively recent evaluation of the instrument in detecting OME (Avery *et al.* 1986) reported a contrary finding. The instrument has been described as diagnostically inferior to the impedance meter (Buhrer *et al.* 1985) but there are recent indications that this view is changing (Schwartz and Schwartz 1987, Oyibohoro *et al.* 1987).

Although not as yet a clinically viable instrument for use with large numbers of children because of the cost and time involved in assessment, auditory brainstem response (ABR) audiometry has also been shown to assist in differentiating conductive losses from sensorineural losses by the pattern of the latency–intensity function (Coats 1978). Using diagnostic testing protocols, it is possible to evaluate the extent of the conductive hearing loss by the displacement of Wave I from the norm at high intensities and by the amount of shift of the latency–intensity function from the norm.

ADVANTAGES AND LIMITATIONS OF IMPEDANCE AUDIOMETRY

Bluestone and Cantekin (1979) summarized the advantages of impedance audiometry as: objectivity; measurement of different parameters than is possible by otoscopy; providing an accurate assessment of middle-ear pressure; and accurate identification of a non-intact tympanic membrane. As already noted, several studies have demonstrated the high degree of specificity and sensitivity of identifying OME by this method.

Its major limitation occurs in the birth to 7 months age-group. The plasticity of the ear canal between these ages may result in artifactual measurements being obtained, as the infant's external auditory meatus does not simulate the hard-walled cavity principles upon which the test is based.

Also, the contralateral acoustic reflex threshold, while yielding a high degree of sensitivity, has been found to have poor specificity (Bluestone *et al.* 1973, Orchik *et al.* 1978, Brooks 1979). Less research has been carried out in the area of ipsilateral acoustic reflexes although recently Marchant *et al.* (1986) reported a finding of high sensitivity (97 per cent) against the results of tympanocentesis, with infants younger than 5 months.

The pathogenesis of OME has been partially attributed to Eustachian tube dysfunction. Immaturity and/or poor muscle function have been suggested as important factors. Clinically, most measures, including impedance audiometry, provide only an indirect assessment of the Eustachian tube function. The Toynbee and Valsalva manoeuvres (see Bluestone 1980) test the ability of the tube to restore middle-ear pressure by swallowing or increasing naso-pharyngeal pressure after negative pressure has been artificially created in the external air canal. More recently, Honjo *et al.* (1984) described a procedure using endoscopic observation of the Eustachian tube.

Pure-tone audiometry

Until the development and widespread use of impedance audiometry, pure-tone audiometry was employed in the majority of investigations of OME. Pure-tone and speech audiometry are still routinely used to assess the degree of hearing loss but they cannot assess the condition of the middle ear. The air-conduction–bone-conduction threshold difference (*i.e.* the air–bone gap) provides a measure of the degree of conductive impairment and is generally only assessed as part of the complete testing protocol once children are old enough to co-operate.

Although normative data have not been obtained on pure-tone thresholds in children, some writers have contended that hearing thresholds in children are higher (*i.e.* better) than thresholds considered as within normal limits for adults (see Bluestone 1983). However, Brooks (1979) reviewed several studies and concluded that younger children have poorer thresholds than older children. As all testing equipment (*e.g.* audiometers, impedance meters) is calibrated according to data based on adult 'audiometric zero' (Martin 1981), it is difficult to assess the real degree of hearing loss attributable to OME in the paediatric population. As OME can result in a hearing loss of from 0 to 60dB HTL, with an average of 15 to 20dB HTL (Bluestone *et al.* 1973, Brooks 1979), it is possible that many children continue to have pure-tone thresholds better than 20 to 25dB HTL in the presence of middle-ear disorders. The value of air-conduction audiometry alone is therefore limited in the identification of children with OME.

Diagnoses would be assisted by the inclusion of bone-conduction thresholds but this requires a higher degree of skill on the part of the tester and of co-operation from the child, and is not generally feasible in patients under about 5 years of age. These tests are unable, therefore, to assess the major proportion of those children between 6 months and 3 years of age who are most at risk for OME. It should be remembered, however, that they were designed to assess hearing levels rather than middle-ear function.

Identification and diagnosis: conclusions

A distinction needs to be made as to which tests are most appropriate to screening, to routine clinical diagnosis, and to research studies—with the highest possible quality of diagnosis being required for the latter. Bluestone and Cantekin (1979) have emphasized the need for each test to be cross-validated to ensure its value in the battery of tests administered. This comment is of particular concern in relation to otomicroscopy, where accuracy is high in expert hands but diminishes rapidly with the less skilled operator. Impedance audiometry follows closely behind otomicroscopy, with test results indicating a high degree of sensitivity and specificity.

Several studies (Orchik *et al.* 1978, Fiellau-Nikolajsen 1980, Renvall *et al.* 1980) have compared tympanograms with findings at myringotomy immediately following that measure. Negative middle-ear pressure ($<-150mmH_2O$), low compliance, reduced gradient or slope of the tympanogram combined with absence of acoustic reflex thresholds were found to be predictive of the state of middle-ear effusion. The amount of fluid was also related to the gradient of the tympanogram —that is, rounded (no clear peak) with fluid up to the umbo level and flattened when the cavity was 'full' of fluid. None of these measures, however, was indicative of hearing loss *per se*, although low compliance measures and amount of fluid in the tympanic cavity have been found to be related to the magnitude of the associated hearing loss (Fiellau-Nikolajsen 1980). There appears to be no significant relationship between the viscosity of the effusion and the degree of hearing loss (Bluestone *et al.* 1973). Felding *et al.* (1984) concluded that tympanograms with a gradient of 0.1 were indicative of OME without major hearing impairment, and suggested that this method be used to separate children with OME into those with and without associated major hearing loss. In contrast, Bluestone *et al.* (1973) reported that at myringotomy, effusions were found almost as frequently in ears with average hearing loss better than 25dB HTL as in those with poorer thresholds. Both groups showed a similar proportion of effusions with high viscosity. However, it has been strongly and repeatedly emphasized that impedance audiometry does not assess hearing thresholds and that the consequences of a mixed or sensorineural hearing loss being missed through an over-reliance on tympanometry would be unacceptable.

In conclusion, the literature suggests that an ideal test protocol for the identification and diagnosis of OME in children should include impedance audiometry and microscopy. Pure-tone audiometry should be added to measure hearing levels in both OME cases and cases of sensorineural hearing loss. The audiological and otological assessment protocols of the Dunedin study conformed to this ideal.

Hearing loss

Reports of the degree of hearing loss said to be associated with OME vary. Brooks (1979), for example, concluded from a review of a number of studies that the degree of hearing loss secondary to OME averaged from 15 to 20dB HTL. From another review of the literature, Berman (1981) concluded that OME produced 'a prolonged mild 15dB loss'. Reichman and Healey (1983), on the other hand, have suggested from their analysis of the literature that losses of from 20 to 30dB HTL are usual, but that for some children the figure may go as high as 50dB HTL. Apparent discrepancies in the hearing loss attributed to OME may reflect differing study populations. Figures obtained from representative populations would be expected to show lesser degrees of hearing loss than figures from hospital clinic populations where hearing loss may be assumed to be a symptom causing the child to be presented to the hospital. Bess (1983) described the typical audiometric profile associated with OME as 'relatively flat, with slight peaking at 2000Hz'. He reported a pure-tone average threshold for the speech frequency range (500, 1000 and 2000Hz) of 27.6dB HTL. He noted, also, that conductive losses of 10dB HTL or more may accompany negative middle-ear pressure, even in the absence of effusion.

More recently, Fria *et al.* (1985) have reported hearing levels for 222 infants, aged from 7 to 24 months, and 540 children, aged from 2 to 12 years, with OME. Average air conduction thresholds of 27dB HTL at 500, 1000 and 4000Hz and 20dB HTL at 2000Hz were recorded for the older children, confirming the profile described by Bess. A pure-tone average threshold of 24.5dB HTL was obtained. This was slightly better than the 27.6dB HTL pure-tone average reported by Bess. A mean speech awareness threshold (SAT) of 24.6dB HTL was obtained for the infants and this was found not to vary significantly with age during the first two years of life. At all ages within this group, infants with unilateral OME responded at lower levels than children with bilateral OME. For the older children, a speech reception threshold (SRT) of 22.7dB HTL was obtained. Fria and associates compared the hearing levels in the better and worse ears of children with unilateral and bilateral OME. They identified a continuum of levels beginning with the better ear of children with unilateral OME (10.9dB HTL), followed by the better ear of those with bilateral OME (21.3dB HTL), the worse ear of those with unilateral OME (22.8dB HTL), and finally the worse ear of those with bilateral OME (31.3dB HTL).

This brief review suggests that hearing losses associated with OME generally average around 15 to 30dB HTL. It is useful to relate these figures to generally accepted levels of hearing impairment. The following scale, provided by Green (1978), relates hearing threshold levels (ISO–1964 standard) to commonly used descriptors of the severity of hearing impairment.

HTL range (dB)	*Degree of impairment*
−10–26	Normal limits
27–40	Mild hearing loss
41–55	Moderate hearing loss
56–70	Moderately severe hearing loss
71–90	Severe hearing loss
91+	Profound hearing loss

According to this scale, the reported hearing threshold levels associated with OME fall largely within 'normal' hearing limits; however, the pure-tone average of

27.6dB HTL reported by Bess (1983), would be classified as mild hearing loss.

Some writers consider that the above scale, which relates to adult hearing threshold levels, may not be relevant for young children. Brooks (1979), for instance, found evidence in several studies that younger children have poorer thresholds than older children. He suggested mean hearing threshold levels of 13, 7 and 5dB for children aged 3, 5 and 7 years respectively. Northern and Downs (1978) proposed that the following scale should be adopted for children learning to talk.

HTL range (dB)	*Degree of impairment*
15–30	Mild hearing loss
31–50	Moderate hearing loss
51–80	Severe hearing loss
81–100	Profound hearing loss

Fria *et al.* (1985), however, compared pure-tone average thresholds for children aged between 2 and 12 years and found no significant differences. Apparent poorer hearing thresholds in younger children may relate more to the child's ability to co-operate while undergoing audiometric testing than to actual differences in hearing levels. The New Zealand Board of Health Committee on Hearing (1984) considered that children with a four-frequency (500, 1000, 2000 and 4000Hz) average hearing threshold level of 15dB or worse should be regarded as suffering from hearing loss.

Developmental consequences

There has been considerable debate in the past 10 to 15 years over the psychological, educational and social consequences of hearing impairment, secondary to OME, in the developing child. A substantial number of studies have been reported during this time, the results of which have generally been interpreted as supporting the view that the fluctuating, mild, conductive hearing losses associated with OME may have deleterious effects on children's speech and language development, intelligence, educational achievement, and behaviour or social and emotional adjustment. Doubt as to the reliability and validity of many of these studies was raised by a small but influential group of writers at the beginning of this decade and since that time other researchers and reviewers have expressed a greater awareness of the methodological problems associated with this research. The overwhelming weight of opinion, nevertheless, continues to support the view that OME and its attendant hearing loss can have deleterious developmental consequences for children suffering from the condition during the first years of life. In the view of those writers most critical of the studies on which this opinion is based, however, the quality of recent research has improved little on earlier work and, therefore, the question remains unresolved. The development of this debate and the current status of knowledge and opinion are surveyed in the following sections.

Early research

The seminal work in this area was conducted in a study reported by Holm and Kunze (1969). In this frequently cited study, the speech and language skills of a group of 16 children with middle-ear disease described as serous or chronic otitis media were compared with those of a matched comparison group of otoscopically normal children with no hearing loss to gross testing. The children in both groups were outpatients of a Seattle orthopaedic hospital, were Caucasian, and were aged between 5½ and 9 years. The two groups were matched for age and sex, and the children in each attended public schools with comparable standards of education. None of the children exhibited obvious mental retardation, conditions associated with retarded development, major congenital anomalies or chronic illness, except in the case of the target group. For these latter children onset of the disease had occurred before 2 years of age, was still present at the time of the study, and had been accompanied by fluctuating hearing levels throughout its duration. At the time of the study the hearing levels of the target group were 'not sufficiently depressed to affect . . . test performance' (Holm and Kunze 1969), while those of the comparison group were normal. The tests administered to the two groups were the Illinois Test of Psycholinguistic Abilities (ITPA), the Peabody Picture Vocabulary Test, the Templin-Darley Picture Articulation Screening Test, and the Mecham Verbal Language Development Scale, a measure of language use in the home (as observed by parents). They found that with the exception of only one subtest of the ITPA the OME group performed significantly ($p \leq 0.05$) worse than the comparison group on all tests requiring 'the receiving or processing of auditory stimuli or the production of a verbal response'. In contrast, the groups performed equally well on tests requiring visual skills with, again, only the one exception. These test findings were confirmed by parents' observations of language use in the home.

In discussing their findings, Holm and Kunze acknowledged that the design of their study may not have controlled for such factors as 'intelligence, environmental stimulation, motivation, and language experience in the home'. Nevertheless, they felt justified in concluding that the evidence of deficiencies on the tests requiring auditory and vocal skills, but not on the tests requiring visual skills, gave strength to the argument that the difference between the two groups was due to the hearing impairment in the OME group.

Throughout the decade which followed this study, an increasing number of researchers reported findings which, in general, confirmed those of Holm and Kunze. This growing literature was reviewed a number of times toward the end of the decade and the view was expressed repeatedly, although not without some reviewers expressing their reservations, that an association existed between OME and deficits in speech and language development, intelligence, educational achievement, and behaviour problems or social and emotional adjustment. Menyuk (1979), for instance, concluded that despite deficiencies in both the quantity and quality of the available literature, 'the data collected thus far indicate that differences in language development do exist'. From a less critical survey of the literature, Mustain (1979) observed that while single or infrequent episodes of middle-ear effusions 'do not seriously compromise language and speech develop ment or educational progress . . . the child with chronic middle ear pathology, particularly during the first three years of life, should be considered at risk' in this regard. A comprehensive review of the studies reported during this period is provided by Rapin (1979). Although cognisant of inadequacies in this literature, Rapin concluded that 'middle ear disease and conductive hearing loss have deleterious consequences for school children's verbal skills and scholastic performance, in particular their reading level'. Finally, in summarizing discussions at a workshop on OM and child development, Ruben and Hanson (1979) concluded that the 'temporary fluctuating mild hearing loss . . . associated with recurrent otitis media, may well have a significant effect' on child development. They suggested that this effect would most likely be subtle, that its primary impact would be on the acquisition of language skills, and that it would have indirect consequences for cognition, social adjustment, school performance, and academic achievement. The research design problems in previous studies were acknowledged by the participants in the workshop who called for a more sophisticated multidisciplinary approach to research on this problem. A number of the more frequently cited studies from this period are reviewed briefly below. It is unfortunate that several of the more influential studies deal with acute OM and not OME (*e.g.* Kaplan *et al.* 1973, Lewis 1976).

Needleman (1977) studied 20 children, aged 3 to 8 years, with a documented history of recurrent OME and fluctuating hearing thresholds and 20 comparison children matched for chronological age, mental age, school grade and socio-economic status. The children in the target group had suffered their first episode of OME before 18 months of age and had experienced recurrent episodes for at least two years. The comparison group had no history of OME or hearing problems. Various phonologic skills were tested, including the production of phonemes (or units of significant sound in a given language) in single words and in connected speech (Templin–Darley Screening Test of Articulation), the discrimination of phonemes (Goldman–Fristoe–Woodcock Test of Auditory Discrimination), the ability to synthesize verbally presented separate sounds into a single word (Sound Blending subtest of the ITPA), the ability to fill in missing speech sounds (Auditory Closure Subtest of the ITPA), and the use of similar combinations of phonemes in different morphologic contexts. Needleman (1977) reported significant differences between the OME and comparison groups in total performance ($p<0.01$), production of phonemes in single words ($p<0.01$) and in connected speech ($p<0.01$), and in the use of similar combinations of phonemes in different morphologic contexts ($p<0.02$). In all of the above cases the comparison group had higher mean scores than the target group. The groups performed equally well on the discrimination task and the Sound Blending and Auditory Closure subtests of the ITPA. By plotting mean performance scores against age, Needleman (1977) was able to show a narrowing gap between the OME and comparison groups as age increased. Needleman speculated from this finding that 'children with early intermittent hearing loss may eventually be able to "catch up" in their phonologic development'.

Whereas the studies reviewed above took groups of children with or without histories of early and recurrent OM and compared their performance on various developmental measures, Masters and Marsh (1978) reported a study which was 'designed to determine the incidence of middle ear pathology in groups of learning disabled and regular class students'. A further aim of this study was to assess the general levels of language functioning in the two groups. The students were selected from elementary schools, were Caucasian, middle class, and had passed a school-administered hearing examination in the year before the study. The learning-disabled students (N=108) had IQs of between 90 and 110 and were impaired in one or more language functions (*i.e.* understanding, reception, organization, expression), while the regular students (N=179) had no 'gross sensory, psychological, or motor problems'. From these students, two groups of 33 were selected on the basis of the results of an impedance audiometry test. One group contained students with B or C type curves, taken to indicate middle-ear pathology, and the other contained students assessed as having normal middle-ear function. No test of hearing levels was reported. The general language function of all 66 students was assessed using the Utah Test of Language Development. Masters and Marsh reported that 12.8 per cent of the 179 regular students and 25 per cent of the 108 learning-disabled students showed evidence of middle-ear pathology ($\chi^2=9.27$, $p<0.01$). Curiously, the only results from the test of language development that Masters and Marsh offered were comparisons between those students with and without middle-ear pathology *within* each condition (regular and learning-disabled), no significant differences being found in either condition. No comparison between conditions was reported. The only conclusion the authors could draw, therefore, was that significantly more learning-disabled students showed evidence of middle-ear pathology at the time of testing. The value of this study is further diminished by the vaguely defined and poorly matched target and comparison groups, and by the loose definition of middle-ear pathology.

Another study which identified the prevalence of OME among learning-disabled children was reported by Freeman and Parkins (1979). In that study 50 children classified as learning-disabled and 32 children who had no apparent learning problems were given an otological examination, and pure-tone and impedance audiometric testing was conducted. The children ranged in age from 6 to 14 years. The clinical examination revealed that 20 per cent of the learning-disabled children compared with 9.5 per cent of the non-learning-disabled group had evidence of OME. Similarly, the pure-tone average for the learning-disabled group was 7.5dB HTL, while that for the comparison group was 3.9dB HTL. Finally, 36 per cent of the learning-disabled children compared with 15.6 per cent of the comparison group had middle-ear pressure more negative than $-100mmH_2O$, and over three times as many learning-disabled children had abnormal tympanograms as did children in the comparison group. No test of the statistical significance of these findings was reported.

Bennett *et al.* (1980) also reported a greater prevalence of chronic OM in learning-disabled children than in controls. They compared two groups of 7- to 12-year-old children matched for age, sex and race. The first group consisted of 53 children who attended full-time language and learning disability classes because of early learning problems and poor performance on achievement, perceptual and language measures. The comparison group consisted of 56 children from regular classes in the same schools as the first group. They had no history of learning problems. The authors found that significantly ($p<0.05$) more of the learning-disabled group (23 per cent) had a history of recurrent OM than did the comparison group (9 per cent). Based on a criterion of a hearing loss of greater than 20dB, 38 per cent of the learning-disabled children had abnormal audiograms while this was true for only 16 per cent of the children in the comparison group. Again, this difference was significant ($p<0.05$). 49 per cent of the learning-disabled group compared with 21 per cent of controls had abnormal tympanograms ($p<0.01$). The authors concluded from their data that while 'a causal relationship between chronic otitis media and school learning problems cannot be inferred . . . the evidence certainly suggests an association between these two disorders.'

Zinkus, Gottlieb and their associates reported a series of studies concerned with the developmental and psycho-educational sequelae of chronic OM. In the first of these studies (Zinkus *et al.* 1978) they compared 18 children who had a history of either chronic OME or recurrent acute OM in the first three years of life, with 22 children who had experienced no more than one brief episode of OM per year during this period. The children, all of whom had been referred to a behavioural paediatric unit because of academic underachievement, ranged in age from 6 to 11 years, were Caucasian, came from middle-class backgrounds, had no history of CNS disease or injury, severe behaviour or emotional disorders, or visual perceptual dysfunctions, and had a Full-scale IQ score which exceeded a criterion value of one standard deviation below the mean. Of those children in the OME or acute OM group, seven had a bilateral hearing loss of 10 to 20dB, six had a unilateral hearing loss of 10 to 20dB, and five had 'auditory acuity within normal limits'. Two of the children in the comparison group had a unilateral hearing loss of 10 to 20dB, while the remainder had 'normal auditory acuity'. Parent interviews and medical records were used to determine the age at which the children had acquired motor, speech and language skills. The WISC-R was used to assess verbal and non-verbal skills and general intelligence, while the Wide Range Achievement Test was used to measure educational performance in the areas of word recognition (decoding), spelling and arithmetic. The personnel administering these tests were unaware of each child's history of OM. The results indicated that, when compared to the controls, the children with chronic or recurrent OM were significantly ($p<0.05$) delayed in speech and language development, had significantly ($p<0.05$) lower Full-scale, Verbal and Performance IQ scores, and scored significantly ($p<0.05$) below expected achievement levels in word recognition and spelling. The groups did not differ, however, with regard to arithmetic skills. In commenting on these findings, the authors drew a parallel between their own work and the study reported by Holm and Kunze (1969). They noted that whereas the earlier study had failed to control for variations in the IQ of the subjects, they had controlled for this factor and, furthermore, had demonstrated that reading ability was not related to intelligence. It must be asked, however, what these authors meant by 'hearing losses of 10 to 20dB' and 'auditory acuity within normal limits', given the difficulty of measuring accurate hearing threshold levels in children.

In the second of these studies (Gottlieb *et al.* 1979) a similar research design to that described above was followed, with, again, children who had been referred for specialist assessment because of 'poor school performance or suspected developmental delays'. Two groups of children were involved in the study. The first consisted of 177 children with 'significant central auditory processing deficits' and the other, 36 children with no evidence of such deficits. Each group was divided into those children with and those without a reported history of chronic or recurrent OM from an early age. A comprehensive battery of measures was obtained for each child, including a behavioural assessment (activity level, attention span, distractibility, impulsivity, anxiety level, motivation and attitude), screening for developmental delays, perceptual weaknesses and academic deficiencies (Physicians Developmental Screening Test), and assessment of intelligence (WISC–R), educational achievement (WRAT), and auditory and visual processing abilities (ITPA). Gottlieb *et al.* reported that 46.3 per cent of those children with 'auditory perceptual disturbances' and 22.2 per cent of those without showed evidence of 'severe chronic otitis media', including 'multiple ear infections during the first three years of life . . . persistent purulent nasal discharge, "draining ears", sinusitis and hearing loss'. This finding was taken as evidence of 'a possible cause for certain types of auditory processing deficits'. They concluded that their data appeared to 'support previous investigations that suggest an association between recurrent middle ear disease, central auditory processing deficits and delayed language development'. They drew similar conclusions in relation to verbal skills, behavioural problems and poor school performance.

In the final study of this series, Zinkus and Gottlieb (1980) attempted to 'determine the effects of chronic otitis media on the pattern and severity of auditory processing deficits'. They again chose children 'referred for evaluation because of academic underachievement' as their subjects. The children were assigned to one of three groups, with 20 subjects in each. Those in Group One had a history of chronic OM during the first three years of life, and had evidence of auditory processing deficits as determined by psychological, speech and language, and educational testing. Just over half had normal hearing at the time of the study, while the remainder had varying degrees of mild to moderate, unilateral or bilateral hearing loss. The children in Group Two had experienced no more than one episode of OM per year during the first three years of life, had been diagnosed as having auditory processing deficits, and most had normal hearing at the time of the study. Two had a mild hearing loss. Finally, those in Group Three had been referred for evaluation but showed no evidence of auditory processing deficits when examined. Five of the children in this group had a mild unilateral or bilateral hearing loss. Groups Two and Three acted as the comparison groups for the study. Parent interviews and medical records were again used to establish the age of acquisition of developmental skills, the WISC-R was used to measure intelligence and verbal and non-verbal skills, and the WRAT to assess educational skills. In addition, the Carrow Test for Auditory Comprehension of Language and the ITPA were used to assess auditory processing ability. The results obtained by Zinkus and Gottlieb indicated that in comparison to Groups Two and Three the children with a history of OM and evidence of auditory processing deficits (Group 1) were significantly ($p<0.05$) slower in developing a 10-word vocabulary and significantly ($p<0.05$) delayed in acquiring three-word phrases. A closer examination of the auditory processing skills of 10 subjects from each group revealed that while both groups with auditory processing deficiencies performed poorly on both the Carrow Test for Auditory Comprehension of Language and the ITPA, those with a history of chronic OM (Group 1) scored significantly lower than Group Three on more subtests of the ITPA than did those without (Group 2). Similarly, the subjects with chronic OM (Group 1) had significantly lower Full-scale, Verbal and Performance IQ scores (all $p<0.01$) than Groups Two and Three. The subjects in Group Two scored significantly lower than Group Three on Full-scale IQ ($p<0.05$) and Verbal IQ ($p<0.01$) but not on Performance IQ. On the test of academic achievement (WRAT), both groups with auditory processing deficits (Groups 1 and 2) scored significantly ($p<0.01$) lower than Group Three in reading, spelling and arithmetic. Groups One and Two differed significantly from each other on reading skills only ($p<0.05$). In discussing these findings Zinkus and Gottlieb concluded that in the particular population with which they were concerned there appeared to be 'a relationship between chronic otitis media in the first three years of life and subsequent deficits in auditory processing, language, and academic skills'. They drew attention specifically to the 'significant delays in the use of three-word phrases' which, they argued, may provide an early indication of 'impending auditory processing difficulties'. With regard to intellectual development they noted that, where tests allowed for repetition of verbal instructions, the chronic OM sufferers performed 'adequately'. This was taken to imply that although cognitive skills might be intact, their use was limited by faulty auditory input, requiring repetition of instructions until these were understood. They speculated, also, that poor performance on some subtests of the WISC (*e.g.* Digit Span, Auditory Sequential Memory) suggested a 'generalised attentional deficit' in those children with a history of OM. Finally, they noted that the most obvious deficits occurred in academic achievement, particularly in the area of reading. They acknowledged, however, that the children assigned to Group One represented 'an extreme on the continuum of chronicity and severity' with regard to OM. They noted that to generalize from this sample to children with OM of lesser severity and chronicity would be inappropriate.

In a departure from most of the studies conducted during this period, Dobie and Berlin (1979) carried out a series of experiments in which they focused on the hearing loss associated with OME. This is, they argued, 'the most obvious link between otitis media and the developmental and educational processes'. They began their investigation by plotting 'the typical frequencies and relative amplitudes for the common speech sounds in English' against the mean hearing levels for people with OME at frequencies ranging from 125 to 8000Hz (both sets of measures expressed in dB SPL). From this analysis they determined that the upper and lower ends of the speech spectrum would be most vulnerable to interference due to a hearing loss of around 20dB. In their first experiment they used a computer simulation technique to determine what acoustic information may be lost to the OM child with a 20dB hearing loss. They concluded that:

1. Morphological markers might be lost or sporadically misunderstood; for example, "Where are Jack's gloves to be placed?" might be perceived as "Where Jack glove be place?".

2. In a related fashion, very short words which are elided often in connected speech (see *"are"* and *"to"* above) will lose considerable loudness because of the critical relationship between intensity, duration, and loudness.

3. Inflections, or markers, carrying subtle nuances such as questioning and related intonation contouring, can at the very best be expected to come through inconsistently.

Similar losses to those predicted were demonstrated by Dobie and Berlin in a second experiment, in which they applied the same computer simulation technique used in the first experiment to auditory confusion actually experienced by a child with chronic OME. This child was found to confuse stops for sibilants 'as both could be perceived as brief silent periods'. From these preliminary findings they concluded that 'one thing that is clear so far is that syllable counts are usually preserved, but microstructure of the articulation (and occasionally markers critical to meaning) may be lost' by children with OME.

CRITICISM OF THE EARLY RESEARCH

In the first major critical review of this research to appear in the literature, Ventry (1980) found that many of the reported studies contained serious 'methodological flaws' and that often the work was poorly documented. Among the methodological flaws he identified were vague subject selection criteria (*e.g.* Masters and Marsh 1978, Needleman 1977), inadequate matching of target and comparison group subjects (*e.g.* Holm and Kunze 1969, Needleman 1977, Masters and Marsh 1978, Zinkus *et al.* 1978), failure to determine the extent of hearing loss at the time of developmental testing (*e.g.* Holm and Kunze 1969, Needleman 1977), lack of control over experimenter bias (*e.g.* Holm and Kunze 1969, Needleman 1977), use of inappropriate tests (*e.g.* Holm and Kunze 1969), failure to randomize or counterbalance test presentations (*e.g.* Needleman 1977), and misinterpretation of test results (*e.g.* Masters and Marsh 1978, Zinkus *et al.* 1978). With regard to the documentation of studies, Ventry observed that some authors had failed to provide information on the validity and reliability of the tests used (*e.g.* Holm and Kunze 1969, Needleman 1977), some had neglected to identify the statistical tests used (*e.g.* Kaplan *et al.* 1973, Zinkus *et al.* 1978), and many had presented a biased interpretation of their findings by emphasizing those results which supported the hypothesized relationship (*e.g.* Kaplan *et al.* 1973, Lewis 1976, Needleman 1977, Zinkus *et al.* 1978).

A second critical appraisal of the studies reviewed above was provided by Paradise (1981; see also Paradise 1980, Paradise and Rogers 1980). The faults which he found in this research included uncertain validity of diagnoses, absence of data on hearing levels in early life, a greater prevalence of hearing impairment in experimental subjects at the time of developmental testing, inadequate matching of target and comparison subjects on variables known to influence development (*e.g.* socio-economic status, environmental stimulation, quality of parenting), biased sampling, small sample sizes, experimenter bias, use of inappropriate tests and selective emphasis in the reporting of results. In addition to questioning the quality of the reported studies, Paradise noted that none had rejected the possibility of there being one or more underlying factors which predispose children to *both* OME and developmental impairments. Possible factors were seen to include low socio-economic status, impaired parenting, subtle unrecognized CNS disorders, and 'conditions that detract from overall health and function, such as recurrent or chronic respiratory infection, or respiratory or other types of allergy'.

Berman (1981), in a third critical review of this literature, also found many of the methodological problems identified by Ventry and Paradise. It is notable that none of these reviewers rejected the possibility of a relationship between OME and developmental delays. Rather, it was their view that none of the studies reviewed had provided conclusive evidence of such a relationship.

Since the publication of those reviews opinion has become divided, with two fairly distinct views emerging. One view accepts the criticisms levelled by Ventry, Paradise and Berman and calls for more and better designed research. The other view acknowledges the inadequacies which exist in the research to date but argues that the weight of evidence does point to a relationship between OME and developmental deficits.

Hignett (1983), for instance, examined 10 of the most frequently cited studies on the effects of OME and, finding methodological problems in each, concluded that 'what is still needed is a sophisticated, well-controlled study to demonstrate a clear connection between OME with transient hearing loss and later developmental impairments'. In contrast, Zinkus (1982) reviewed many of the same studies and, while acknowledging problems associated with them, concluded that 'the results of these investigations . . . do suggest a possible association between the delayed acquisition of speech and language, auditory processing disturbances, and early severe otitis media during the first 3 years of life'. A similar conclusion was drawn by Zinkus in regard to the effects of OME on academic achievement. The same acknowledgement of methodological flaws in research appeared in a review by McDermott (1983) but, again, the conclusion was reached that 'middle ear disease causes irreversible physical and developmental changes in the young child'. Similarly, in a recent and comprehensive review by Reichman and Healey (1983), it was concluded that 'sufficient data have been presented to suggest that children with early onset, recurrent otitis media and mild hearing loss may be at risk for developing delays in auditory, language, and academic skills'. These authors divided the literature into two groups, those examining children with a history of early OME and current hearing impairment and those examining children with early-onset resolved OME and normal hearing. They concluded from the first group of studies that it was impossible to determine whether observed developmental delays were due to '*current* or *historic* auditory deprivation'. From their review of studies in the second group, they observed that none had 'found otitis-prone groups to lack a pattern of depressed performance and statistically significant gaps' on the developmental tests used. Similarly, Downs (1982, 1983) pointed to the sheer volume of research which has found a relationship between OME and developmental deficits and observed that 'no amount of cavilling over experimental design can obviate the fact that serious attention must be given to these findings' (Downs 1983). She reviewed two comparatively recent studies (Sak and Ruben 1981, Teele *et al.* 1981) in which attempts had been made to avoid some of the methodological problems of earlier studies, and found further evidence in these of a relationship between OME and developmental delays. Finally, both

Ventry (1983) and Paradise (1983) commented on research appearing in the literature since their first critical reviews. Ventry said he could find nothing in this more recent work to change his original opinion that 'no causal link has been established between early recurrent middle ear effusion and any behavioural phenomenon of interest'. Furthermore, he expressed concern that there had been no apparent advances in research design since the early work of Holm and Kunze (1969). He then advanced several ways in which research could be improved, including the abandonment of between-subject retrospective designs, the greater use of both experimental and descriptive within-subject designs (including longitudinal studies), the increased use of correlational designs, and much greater attention to factors threatening the internal validity of studies. Paradise (1983) reviewed four recent studies (Sak and Ruben 1981, Hoffman-Lawless *et al.* 1981, Teele *et al.* 1981, Friel-Patti *et al.* 1982) and, like Ventry, reaffirmed his opinion that 'no convincing evidence currently exists that adverse developmental consequences result from otitis media limited to the first few years of life'. He too made an urgent call for 'appropriately designed studies', giving as his reasons the lack of contrary evidence and the prevalence of the disease.

Recent research

The purpose of this final section is to review the studies which have appeared in the literature since 1980. While a number of these will have been conducted prior to the critical reviews of Ventry (1980), Berman (1981) and Paradise (1981), those reported more recently, at least, should reflect the increased awareness by researchers of the methodological problems associated with this area of research. Several of these studies were referred to in the reviews by Downs (1983) and Paradise (1983) but a number are relatively recent contributions to current knowledge on the relationship between OME and child development.

Brandes and Ehinger (1981) reported a study in which they examined the effects of early middle-ear pathology on auditory and visual perceptual skills, academic achievement and non-verbal intelligence. Their subjects were 30 schoolchildren of approximately 8 years of age, sampled from a predominantly middle-class suburban population in British Columbia. One half of the children had in the previous year failed a pure-tone screening test (20dB HTL at 1000, 2000 and 4000Hz) and had a history of middle-ear problems in the first three years of life. Matched with these subjects were 15 children sampled from the same population, but who had passed the screening test in the previous year and had no significant history of middle-ear problems between birth and the time of the study. The battery of tests administered to the children included the Goldman–Fristoe–Woodcock Auditory Skills Test Battery, the Peabody Individual Achievement Test, the Wide Range Achievement Test, the Motor-Free Visual Perception Test and the Ravens Coloured Progressive Matrices. Before those tests were administered, the speech reception thresholds of the children in both groups were measured. The mean threshold for the target group was 12dB HTL and that for the comparison group 7dB HTL. An analysis of variance conducted on the combined test scores indicated a significant difference between the two groups ($F=10.49$, $p<0.05$). When the separate test scores were analysed, however, only the Selective

Attention subtest of the Auditory Skills Test Battery showed a significant difference between the two groups. Although Brandes and Ehinger made much of the poorer performance of the target group on most of the tests administered, it is apparent from the results of their analyses that the two groups differed only on tasks involving the discrimination of auditory stimuli under conditions of background noise. Given the difference in speech reception thresholds for the two groups this result is perhaps unsurprising, although the difference was only 5dB HTL and both groups fell within the normal limits for speech reception thresholds at the time of testing. Of greater significance was the finding that the two groups did not differ at 8 years of age on the tests of academic achievement. Weaknesses in this study included vague subject selection procedures and reliance on the otological history and current audiological status of children for group assignment. Otological history, based on parent reports, is generally considered to be the least reliable indicator of middle-ear disease and current audiological status tells nothing of the child's ability to hear during the critical speech and language learning period up to the age of 5 or 6 years.

Another study which examined the effects of early onset OME on auditory processing abilities was reported by Hoffman-Lawless *et al.* (1981). Four groups of 10 children participated in the study, two with an average age of 7 years and two with an average age of 9 years. One group at each age consisted of children who had acquired OME before the age of 4 years and had had tympanostomy tubes inserted before their fifth birthday. The children in the other two groups had no known history of OME. The subjects in all four groups had normal hearing and middle-ear function at the time of the study. That is, they had hearing thresholds between 0 and 15dB in the speech frequencies, speech discrimination scores better than 88 per cent at 30dB SPL (sound pressure level), middle-ear pressure between 0 and $-200mmH_2O$, static compliance between 0.3 and $1.5cm^3$ of equivalent volume of air, and acoustic reflex thresholds of less than 95dB HTL at 500, 1000 and 2000Hz. The authors found that the 7-year-old OME group scored significantly lower ($F=4.09$, $df=1, 36$, $p<0.01$) on a filtered speech test than the control group at this age. There was no significant difference between the 9-year-old groups on this test. No significant differences were obtained between groups at either age on the Staggered Spondaic Word Test, a speech-in-noise test, the auditory sequential memory test from the ITPA or the sound-blending test of the Goldman–Fristoe–Woodcock Auditory Skills Test Battery. Hoffman-Lawless *et al.* concluded from these findings that their study had failed to identify a clear link between a history of OME exceeding nine months in children aged 4 years or less who were adequately treated and the presence of disordered auditory processing abilities. They commented that the one significant finding they did obtain 'was not clinically meaningful and would not be considered as having implications for auditory language learning'. The finding that this difference was not present in the 9-year-olds suggested to them that delays in auditory processing abilities may be temporary rather than permanent. While this study may be criticized both for its small group sizes and for the lack of any attempt to match subjects other than for age and sex, it was methodologically sound in most other respects. As the authors suggested, auditory processing defects may be more likely to occur in children who acquire OME at a younger age than did those in their study. Moreover, they suggested that 'children who receive effective medical or surgical care . . . may be less apt to acquire disorders of central auditory abilities, since their conductive hearing loss is minimised'.

An interesting method of matching subjects was used in a study reported by Sak and Ruben (1981). 18 pairs of siblings between the ages of 8 and 11 years participated in this study, one sibling in each pair having a history of OME and the other having no history of the disease. The children were given comprehensive pure-tone and impedance evaluations, plus an otological examination, a complete medical history was obtained, and a battery of psychological and educational tests were administered. The latter test battery included the WISC–R, Ravens Coloured Progressive Matrices, the ITPA, the WRAT and the Durrell Analysis of Reading Difficulty. The siblings with a history of OME had experienced their first episode during their first four years of life and all had had tympanostomy tubes inserted by their fourth birthday. At the time of testing, all subjects had bilateral or unilateral pure-tone average hearing thresholds of 15dB HTL or less and speech reception thresholds of 10dB HTL or less. All had normal speech discrimination ability. 50 per cent of the OME siblings had abnormal impedance results at the time of testing compared to 22 per cent of the control subjects. From their analysis of the psychological and educational test data, Sak and Ruben found that the mean Full-scale IQs (WISC–R) of both groups were in the above-average range, that the groups did not differ on this measure, on Performance IQ, or on the measure of Non-verbal Intelligence (Raven), but that the OME group had a significantly lower mean Verbal IQ than the comparison group (111 versus 116). There was no significant difference between the groups on nine out of the 11 subtests of the ITPA but the OME group scored significantly lower than the comparison group on the Auditory Reception subtest and significantly higher on the Visual Sequential Memory subtest. The groups did not differ significantly on any of the subtests of the WRAT but the OME group was significantly below actual grade placement in spelling achievement. Finally, there was no difference between groups on the test of reading comprehension. Sak and Ruben concluded that their results showed minimal deficits secondary to recurrent OME in the preschool years. In commenting on the differences between groups they speculated that the lower Verbal IQ and corresponding higher visual sequential memory scores of the OME group may have indicated 'a compensatory shift in the cognitive strategy of these subjects'. They argued, furthermore, that the 'more pervasive deficits' found in other studies may have resulted from the subjects in those studies being less intellectually and socio-economically advantaged than the subjects in their own study, and therefore less able to develop strategies to compensate for their hearing loss. In his review of Sak and Ruben's report, Paradise (1983) noted that the 'so-called' deficits found in the study may simply have been due to the greater prevalence of minor middle-ear abnormalities in the OME group at the time of the study. Even if this explanation were incorrect, it is clear that Sak and Ruben's findings are not greatly at variance with those of Brandes and Ehinger (1981) and Hoffman-Lawless *et al.* (1981), who found little evidence of long-term developmental deficits resulting from OME occurring during the first five years of life.

In contrast to the preceding studies, Jerger *et al.* (1983) investigated the effects of OM on development in children aged from 2 to 5 years. Two groups of 25 children participated in this study. One group consisted of children with a history of recurrent episodes of OM, the onset of which had occurred between the ages of 2 weeks and 36 months. The average number of episodes for this group was seven per year, and 18 of these children had received surgical treatment for the disease. The control group consisted of 25 children who had received regular otoscopic examination and had no history of OM, frequent respiratory infections or allergy. A comprehensive battery of tests designed to assess speech intelligibility was administered, including measures of verbal ability, non-verbal skills and social maturity. Jerger *et al.* noted that not all of their subjects completed the rigorous testing session which lasted for approximately one-and-a-half hours. Others could not be tested because of the presence of tympanostomy tubes. For these and other reasons the data collected in the study were incomplete on a number of measures. Given the small sample size that the researchers began with (N=50) and the fatiguing battery of tests administered to the children, the results reported by these authors must be interpreted with some caution. The mean hearing threshold levels of the two groups did not differ significantly, with the levels at 1000Hz being 14dB HTL for both the OM and comparison groups. The two groups differed significantly, however, on the measures of verbal skills (Peabody Picture Vocabulary Test and Verbal Language Development Scale) and social maturity (Vineland Social Maturity Scale). On these tests the OM group showed a mean delay in comparison with the control group of five months in vocabulary skills (PPVT), eight months in language skills (VLDS) and five months in social maturity (VSMS). The groups did not differ on the measure of non-verbal skills (Southern California Figure Ground Visual Perception Test). The authors provided a detailed analysis of data collected on the Paediatric Speech Intelligibility (PSI) test. This test consists of word and sentence messages composed by normal children, presented to subjects either in quiet or in competition. In the quiet conditions both groups of children obtained perfect scores for both words and sentences. This was true across all age-groups and was interpreted by the authors as indicating that the children in both groups had both the vocabulary and the cognitive skills to perform the PSI task. Inter-group differences were apparent, however, in the competition condition, where a competing message was presented to the subject. Whereas the children in the comparison group demonstrated an improvement in word scores of 60 per cent from 24 to 30 months of age, those in the OM group improved by only 10 per cent between 2 and 3 years of age. The comparison group reached the ceiling for the test at 36 to 38 months of age while the OM group reached it at the later age of 39 to 47 months. In contrast, for sentences presented in competition, there was no significant difference between groups. In examining their data for an explanation of this result Jerger *et al.* could find no significant relationships between PSI words in competition scores and other variables they had measured, including vocabulary, language ability, social maturity, sex, age of onset of OM, number of episodes per year, and presence or absence of tympanostomy tubes. Seeking an explanation in previous theoretical writings, they turned to work by Dobie and Berlin (1979) and Menyuk (1980) which, they suggested, had anticipated their results. Dobie and Berlin, it will be recalled, concluded from their research on simulated hearing loss that while syllable counts are usually preserved, the microstructure of articulation may be lost to the child with OME-related hearing loss. Jerger *et al.* interpreted this conclusion as meaning that there is 'degradation of acoustic–phonetic information important to word understanding, but preservation of the global information important to sentence comprehension'. This would explain the observed differences between single-word reproduction and sentence reproduction. Menyuk's observations on word discrimination may be taken as support for this view. She argued that while there is a marked improvement in word reproduction between 2 and 4 years of age, 'children three years and older have difficulty in discriminating between two words if they don't know the meaning of the words'. Presumably, when heard in the context of a complete sentence, the meaning of single words will be more apparent, thereby overcoming problems of discrimination. In concluding their report, Jerger *et al.* made no mention of the delays in vocabulary, language skills and social maturity displayed by their OME group. These findings may, however, provide some evidence that OME has an impact during the years in which development is greatest in these particular areas.

Being aware of the criticism levelled at past research and, in particular, 'retrospective' studies, Teele *et al.* (1984) conducted what they described as a 'prospective' study of 205 children aged 3 years. The subjects were selected from among infants enrolled in five Greater Boston health centres at birth and who had received regular otoscopic examinations during their first three years of life. Selection was made on the basis of number of episodes of OME. The socio-economic status (SES) of the children was measured, and a battery of tests of speech and language development were administered, including measures of comprehension (Peabody Picture Vocabulary Test), receptive and expressive language (Zimmerman Pre-school Language Scale), and reproduction of speech sounds (Fisher–Logemann–Goldman–Fristoe Test of Articulation). These tests were administered blind. A screening audiogram was used to determine that no child was sufficiently hearing impaired to be excluded from the sample at the time of testing. Teele *et al.* found that the total duration of OME experienced by their subjects ranged from zero to more than 500 days in three years. The mean total time spent with OME was 116.3 days. The total sample was then divided into three groups based on total time spent with OME—that is, less than 30 days, 30 to 129 days, and 130 or more days. No indication was given of how many children in the less than 30 days group had never had OME. The subjects were further divided into those with high SES or low SES. For the high SES group, scores on the PPVT and on the Auditory Comprehension and Verbal Ability subtests of the Zimmerman Pre-school Language Scale correlated negatively with total time spent with OME during the first three years of life. The correlation coefficients ranged from –0.14 to –0.45, and all but one were significant ($p<0.05$). No significant correlations were obtained for the low-SES group, which led the authors to conclude that SES was an 'important confounding variable'. They then conducted a series of multiple regression analyses, with SES, whether OME was unilateral or bilateral, sex, total time spent with OME, and time when OME occurred as predictor variables, and the various psychological and educational test scores as dependent variables. As expected, SES was found to make a consistent and significant contribution to the multiple regression models. These analyses revealed, in addition, that total time spent with OME, whether it was unilateral or bilateral, and occurrence during the first year—and more especially the first six months—of life, all contributed significantly to the lower test scores on the measures of vocabulary, auditory comprehension and verbal ability. Sex, birth order and pattern of day care were rejected as explanatory variables.

In a follow-up report of this study, Klein *et al.* (1984) presented the results of multiple comparisons performed on their data. For the full sample of 205 children only one significant difference between groups was obtained: children who had had OME for 130 days or more during their first three years of life scored significantly lower on the PPVT than those who had had the disease for less than 30 days ($p<0.05$). When subgroups of high-SES children were compared, however, 'significant' differences were obtained between the under 30 days group and the 30 to 129 days group on the measures of comprehension ($p=0.07$) and verbal ability ($p<0.05$). Significant differences were obtained for the measures of vocabulary ($p<0.01$), comprehension ($p<0.01$) and verbal ability ($p<0.01$), when the under 30 days and over 130 days groups were compared. No such differences were obtained when low SES groups were compared.

In summary, the study reported by Teele *et al.* (1984) and Klein *et al.* (1984) identified a negative association between duration of OME and performance on measures of vocabulary, comprehension and verbal ability. However, this association was found only for those children in the high-SES group, as defined by Teele *et al.* (1984). That is, children in the high-SES group who had OME for between 30 and 129 days performed less well on the measures of comprehension and verbal ability than children in the high-SES group who had OME for less than 30 days. Further, high-SES children who had OME for 130 days or more did not perform as well on the measures of vocabulary, comprehension and verbal ability, as did those high-SES children who had OME for less than 30 days. Children in the low-SES group were not affected in this way.

Teele, Klein and their colleagues expressed confidence that their study avoided most of the deficiencies found in earlier research. They acknowledged, however, that their sampling procedure was not random, and it is in this respect that the greatest criticism can be levelled at their work. To begin with, no attempt was made to substantiate the claim that 'the children studied were similar to the majority of children in the United States and Canada'. The pool of infants from which their sample was drawn included only children attending selected health care centres and not the total population of newborn infants in the geographical area concerned. How this pool of subjects related to the total population of newborn infants in the United States and Canada, or Greater Boston for that matter, was not stated. Secondly, the observations during the three years from birth were made unsystematically in that they were made only when children visited the health centres. The measures of occurrence and duration of the disease may, therefore, have been quite inaccurate and may explain the failure to find significant associations or inter-group differences for the low-SES children. It may be that the parents of these children did not make the same use of the health centres as those in the high-SES group. Finally, while Klein *et al.* (1984) reported significant intergroup differences, they offered no comparison with children having no history of OME. The seriousness of this omission is debatable. On the one hand it might be argued that these researchers, like many others before them, have failed to demonstrate that children affected by OME in early childhood are significantly disadvantaged developmentally in comparison to children with no early history of OME. On the other hand, however, they have demonstrated that an increase in the duration of OME is accompanied by a significant decline in language development. Given the high incidence of OME during early childhood, it may be unrealistic to expect researchers to find a comparison group completely free of OME. The approach taken by Teele, Klein and their associates may be the most that can be achieved in such studies.

The prevalence of OME in a cohort of 387 7-year-old Danish children (Lous and Fiellau-Nikolajsen 1981) was referred to earlier. Lous (1986) has summarized subsequent investigations of the language development of this cohort. The children were assessed using a phonological sentence repetition test. While a variety of background measures such as age, sex, number of siblings and years of day care outside the home were found to be related to phonological development, there was no evidence of a relationship between phonological development and history of OME. There was no evidence either of a relationship between current hearing threshold levels and phonological development. A significant relationship was, however, obtained between phonological development and current middle-ear status as determined by impedance audiometry. Children with bilateral B tympanograms were found to have slightly lower scores on the phonological test.

Lous and Fiellau-Nikkolajsen (1984*a,b*) gave a sample of 523 3-year-olds repeated impedance audiometric tests over a six-month period. Five years later they measured the reading ability of the children using a silent reading test. 31 of those children who had had abnormal (B or C_2 type) tympanograms in at least one ear at each of the four tests administered at 3 years were matched for race, sex, age and social stratum with control subjects from the same school classroom. The control subjects had had bilateral type A tympanograms when tested at the age of 3 years. The authors found that the children with abnormal tympanograms at 3 years did not score significantly differently from the matched comparison group on the silent reading test administered at 8 years.

With regard to the middle-ear status of the children during the five-year period between the impedance audiometry and the reading test, Lous and Fiellau-Nikolajsen (1984*a*) reported that 73 per cent of the abnormal group still had abnormal tympanograms at 6 years of age. The middle-ear status of the control group at this age was not reported but Lous and Fiellau-Nikolajsen found that 48 per cent of those tympanometrically normal ears in the full sample at 3 years were still normal when tested at age 6 years. 18 per cent of these ears were abnormal at the age of 6 years and 32 per cent were not tested.

Given that the incidence of OME is believed to remain relatively high during the mid-childhood years (see p. 5), it is possible that a substantial number of the control-group children in Lous and Fiellau-Nikolajsen's study experienced OME during the five-year period referred to above. If this were so, then comparing the two groups on the silent reading test might be expected to produce the non-significant difference that was obtained. The validity of this comparison must therefore be questioned.

A second comparison, between those children in the sample with abnormal tympanograms at age 3 and a control group of same-sex classmates, produced a similar result to the case–control comparison reported above. In this instance, Lous and Fiellau-Nikolajsen had only limited knowledge of the middle-ear status of the control group at age 3 years and during the intervening five years, and so again the validity of the comparison must be questioned.

In a summary of the above studies and of related research conducted by himself and his colleagues, Lous (1986) drew two major conclusions. First, in reference to the association found between present or recent OME and language development, he suggested that this was 'so slight' as to have 'no practical implications'. Second, he argued that developmental impairments resulting from earlier hearing losses, secondary to OME, are reversible when hearing is restored either spontaneously or following treatment.

The members of a birth cohort of Apache Indian children were assigned by Fischler *et al.* (1985) to one of four groups, on the basis of their history of OM 'attacks'. An attack was defined as a clinical diagnosis of either acute suppurative OM, serous OM or chronic OM. The children were aged from 6 to 8 years at the time of the study, and of the 318 in the original cohort, 175 were included in the study. The groups ranged from 'high risk/recurrent' for those having at least two attacks of OM before their second birthday and at least three attacks since, to 'not high risk/not recurrent' for those having fewer than two attacks before their second birthday and fewer than three since. Two receptive and two expressive language tests (Test of Language Development), an informal measure of articulation, and a measure of non-verbal intelligence (Block Design subscale of the WISC–R) were administered to the children by two speech pathologists who were unaware of the individual histories of OM. The four groups were found not to differ significantly on any of the tests. Moreover, when children with the poorest language performance were compared with those performing best, no significant difference was found in the number of OM attacks experienced by the groups. Children observed to have otological abnormalities just before language testing were found to have significantly lower scores on the Picture Vocabulary, Grammatic Completion and Oral Vocabulary subtests of the Test of Language Development.

While the findings reported by Fischler *et al.* (1985) are generally contrary to the prevailing opinion that OME has deleterious effects on speech and language development, there are many problems associated with this study. The first of these and the one which most limits the usefulness of the study is the method of group assignment. Episodes of acute suppurative OM, serous OM or chronic OM all qualified as OM attacks for this purpose. Since no attempt was made to distinguish between these three types, it is impossible to know if episodes of serous otitis media (OME) had any effect on the language development of the cohort. The authors themselves acknowledged other problems associated with the study. Several physicians were involved in examining the children but no measure of inter-observer reliability was obtained. Examination was dependent on the children being presented at the clinic, a potential source of bias. The duration of attacks and the degree of hearing loss associated with each was not recorded. The language testing was performed in English but this was not the first language of many of the children. Given these problems, it is difficult to see how any useful conclusion can be drawn from this study.

Another study which adds little to the debate is that reported by Van Cauwenberge *et al.* (1985, 1986*b*). The subjects in this study were 1512 'apparently healthy' Belgian infants aged from 25 to 80 months. Speech, language development and 'psycho-intellectual' development were judged on an arbitrary three-point scale, ranging from good through poor to bad, by their infant school teacher 'in cooperation with a sociologist'. Although not stated, the recording of a type B tympanogram appears to have been taken as evidence of OME. The authors presented evidence of 'highly significant' differences between groups, and in their conclusions were adamant that their findings fully justified the practice of early detection and treatment of OME. This study, as reported, appears to have little scientific merit. To begin with, it fails to meet the basic requirement of replicability. Further, no evidence is presented regarding the validity and reliability of the measures used. Finally, the teachers who made the above judgements could not be blind to the medical history of the children, thereby introducing a confounding factor into the design of the study.

Golz (1986) also has reported the findings of a study which, because of inadequacies in design and analysis, contributes little to the present debate. 80 Israeli children, aged from 6 to 8 years, were selected from those attending an outpatient clinic because of recurrent episodes of acute OM or persistent OME. These children were found on repeated testing to have hearing losses in excess of 20dB. A matched control group of 80 children with no history of OM and with normal hearing was also selected. A 'special reading test' was administered to both groups. The study group made significantly more mistakes on this test than did the control group. The percentage of mistakes made on the reading test by the study group was said to be correlated with both the level of hearing loss and the number of ear infections experienced by the children but no correlation coefficients were reported. The percentage of mistakes made by the control group was also said to be correlated with the level of hearing loss (or more correctly, hearing threshold level). This unexpected finding casts real doubt on the validity of the reading test, the nature of which was not described. This omission, the failure to distinguish between acute OM and OME, and the lack of sophistication in the statistical analyses, suggest that little weight should be given to the findings of this study.

A further addition to the growing list of studies which have failed to find a relationship between early onset OME and later language and academic performance has been provided by Roberts *et al.* (1986). In this study, the health status of 61 socio-economically disadvantaged Black children who had entered a day-care programme between the ages of 6 weeks and 3 months was monitored almost daily until they reached the age of 5 years. Diagnosis of OME was made by means of pneumatic otoscopy, with verification by impedance audiometry. Episodes of OME were monitored regularly and the duration of each was recorded. Several standardized tests of intelligence (Stanford–Binet Intelligence Scale,

McCarthy Scale of Children's Abilities, Wechsler Preschool and Primary Scale of Intelligence) and academic achievement (Peabody Individualized Achievement Test) were administered to the children between the ages of 3 and 5 years. The tests were administered blind. To test the hypothesis that 'both unilateral and bilateral OME could alter speech and language perception and detrimentally affect the learning of verbal skills', the total duration of OME experienced during the first three years of life was calculated for each child. No significant correlations were obtained between total duration of OME and scores on any of the tests of intelligence and academic achievement. The children were assigned to one of three groups based on total duration of OME (less than 88 days; 88 to 181 days; more than 181 days). Several multivariate tests were applied to the data. No significant differences between the groups were revealed on any of the measures. Neither was there any evidence of differences between groups in the pattern of change in IQ scores over time.

An important feature of the above study was the close monitoring of the health of each member of the cohort throughout the early childhood years. This allowed for greater precision in measuring each child's total experience of OME. As the authors noted, many previous studies had used the number of episodes of OME as a measure of total experience (*e.g.* Jerger *et al.* 1983, Fischler *et al.* 1985). Given the transient nature of OME, this can be a very inaccurate measure. The design of this study has a number of similarities to that used by Teele *et al.* (1984) and Klein *et al.* (1984). The findings parallel those obtained for the low-SES group in the earlier study but not those for the high-SES group. The children observed by Roberts *et al.* were from a socio-economically disadvantaged group. The debate over comparison groups applies also to this study.

The most recent study to present evidence contrary to the hypothesis that OME is related to poor academic achievement has been reported by Brooks (1986, 1987). In this study the academic attainment levels of 64 young adults were obtained from school reports, interviews and questionnaires. All the subjects had commenced their early education at the same school in 1968 or 1969, and as part of an investigation into OME had undergone repeated impedance testing. No significant correlations were obtained between the measures of OME and academic attainment. As part of this study Brooks (1987) examined time lost from school because of OME and found that, although those children with the disease tended to have more time off school, this factor was unrelated to later academic attainment.

To conclude this review, two studies which involved an alternative approach to the present question will be examined. In these studies, children with developmental disorders were examined for evidence of OME. Eaton and Nowell (1983) tested two groups of London children, aged from 7 to 11 years, for evidence of OM. The first of these groups consisted of 55 children from remedial reading centres, while the second group consisted of 59 children from a normal school. Impedance testing revealed that 14 of the children in the remedial reading group had type B or type C tympanograms, compared with four children in the control group. Chi-square analysis showed that this result was significant. The contrast between the groups was less dramatic, however, when only those children with type B tympanograms were considered. Six children in the remedial group had type B tympanograms, compared with two in the control group. This difference was not significant.

In the second of these studies, Bishop and Edmundson (1986) compared a group of 69 language-disordered children with two control groups matched for age, sex and educational background. The children in all three groups lived in the North East or North West of England. A comprehensive parental questionnaire sought information on perinatal and neurological risk factors, history of ear infections and family history of language disorder. When the groups were compared, the language-disordered group did not differ from the controls with regard to the mean number of episodes of OME experienced. They were, however, significantly over-represented among those children referred for specialist ENT care or who were reported to have undergone surgery for OME. In seeking an explanation for this latter finding, Bishop and Edmundson speculated on the possibility that referral for specialist care was more likely to occur in cases where a child presented with both OME and a language disorder, than in cases where only OME was diagnosed.

Bishop and Edmundson also assessed the language-disordered children on a battery of language tests. Those with and without OME were compared and were found not to differ in either the severity or pattern of language impairment or in respect to prognosis. Bishop and Edmundson did, however, find that children in the language-disordered group with OME had significantly higher scores on a scale of perinatal and neurological risk than did those without OME. They concluded that while OME alone 'may not be a crucial determinant of language disorder, it may interact with other risk factors, so that it becomes important if the child is already vulnerable because of a hazardous perinatal history'. This view is supported by Paden *et al.* (1987) who found in a study of 3-year-olds with frequent or recurring OME that phonologic delay could not be attributed to any single factor such as duration of OME or severity of hearing impairment.

In summary, neither of the above studies produced evidence that OME alone has an aetiological role in developmental language disorders. There is evidence, however, that in combination with other risk factors OME may contribute to developmental deficits.

Conclusions

It is clear from the studies reviewed above that researchers in this field have yet to overcome the many methodological problems identified by Ventry (1980), Berman (1981) and Paradise (1981). The findings of several of these studies have been rejected, or at least viewed sceptically, because of deficiencies found in the methods used.

Most of these studies were concerned with testing for developmental deficits in children who had suffered from OME during their first years of life. Of those studies for which no serious methodological problems were apparent, none were able to present convincing evidence of a causal link between early-onset OME and later developmental deficits. Among these were the studies by Hoffman-Lawless *et al.* (1981) and Sak and Ruben (1981), who found evidence of lower Verbal IQ among children with an early history of OME but described the difference as minimal.

A major difficulty faced in interpreting the findings of those two studies is that all of the subjects concerned had received surgical treatment following identification of the disease. Since in neither study were developmental measures administered prior to intervention, it is impossible to know whether the later lack of evidence of developmental delays was the result of subjects 'catching up' with their unaffected peers after intervention or simply to a lack of impairment before the intervention. The evidence presented by Jerger *et al.* (1983) of delayed vocabulary, impaired language skills, and social immaturity among children aged from 2 to 5 years would tend to support the first of these two interpretations (*i.e.* that children had caught up). It is clear that further research is needed to clarify these issues. Moreover, it is quite apparent, given the failure of almost two decades of research to reach a conclusion acceptable to all, that a fresh approach to the problem is required.

One approach for which there has been considerable support in the literature is that of longitudinal research, in which developmental measures are administered at intervals from the time of identification until the time at which speech and language skills are normally well established (Holm and Kunze 1969, Menyuk 1979, Rapin 1979, Hoffman-Lawless *et al.* 1981, Jerger *et al.* 1983, Hall and Hill 1986). Other writers have identified some of the difficulties associated with longitudinal research. Ventry (1980), for instance, pointed out that 'true experimental work is nearly impossible' in this area. The difficulty, he argued, lies in the fact that 'researchers simply cannot manipulate (that is, induce) hearing impairment on human subjects and then study the effects of that manipulation on behaviour or function'. Hignett (1983) cited the unreliability of language measures, attrition rates and cost as difficulties associated with longitudinal studies.

Despite the above problems, the longitudinal design of the present study was selected as being well suited to the investigation of the assumed developmental consequences of OME. The Dunedin longitudinal study to be described in the ensuing chapters represents a fresh approach to the vital question as to whether or not OME is associated with developmental disadvantage in children and if so, for how long.

2
METHODS

An important advantage of this study was that it provided the opportunity to examine the occurrence of OME in Dunedin children from a longitudinal perspective. In addition, the multidisciplinary nature of the wider study enabled the investigation of a variety of possible antecedents of OME, as well as the developmental and behavioural consequences of the disease.

Subjects

The sample was drawn from a cohort of 1661 infants born at the Queen Mary Hospital between 1 April 1972 and 31 March 1973 to mothers from the Dunedin metropolitan area. Dunedin is the major city of the province of Otago in the south of the South Island of New Zealand and at the time the sample was born had a population of about 110,000. Of the original 1661 infants, 1037 (536 boys and 501 girls) were assessed as 3-year-olds and a high percentage of these were assessed at the ages of 5, 7, 9 and 11 years. Those not assessed at 3 years comprised 12 who had died, 510 who could not be traced or were known to be living beyond the province of Otago, 34 who were traced but too late for inclusion in the sample, and 68 for whom parental co-operation was not obtained. A comparison of the 1037 children assessed as 3-year-olds with the 624 not assessed indicated that they did not differ in terms of prenatal, birth or neonatal characteristics (Silva *et al.* 1981).

The first assessment of the children, at birth, is identified as Phase I of the study. The follow-up assessments, at ages 3, 5, 7, 9 and 11 years, are identified as Phases III, V, VII, IX and XI respectively. These assessments were conducted on, or as close as possible to the child's birthday at each phase.

Table 2.1 shows the number of children assessed and not assessed at each phase of the study. At Phase III all the children were assessed by staff at the study centre. In subsequent phases a majority of the children were assessed at the study centre but some were seen at school or at home and others were assessed elsewhere in the country by members of the Department of Education's Psychological Service. Children not assessed at each phase included those who had died, some who had moved beyond the province of Otago and were not seen, and others for whom parental co-operation had been withdrawn (*i.e.* refusals).

Representativeness of the sample

From a comparison made with total population figures for New Zealand (Silva *et al.* 1981), the sample at Phase III was found to be slightly biased in terms of the Elley and Irving (1972, 1976) Index of Socio-economic Status (SES), having a greater proportion from the highest SES levels and less from the lower levels. There was also a lower proportion of children born to unmarried mothers than in the country as a whole. Finally, the sample was found to be under-representative of children of Maori or other Polynesian extraction, only 2 per cent of the sample being from this group compared with about 10 per cent for the total population of New Zealand.

TABLE 2.1
The sample at each phase of the study*

Phase	*Children assessed*			*Children not assessed*		
	Place seen	*N*		*Reason*	*N*	
III	Study centre	1037				
V	Study centre	917		Not seen	33	
	School or home	22		Refusals	12	
	Psych. service	52		Died	1	
	Total	991	(96%)	Total	46	(4%)
VII	Study centre	877		Not seen	51	
	School or home	14		Refusals†	30	
	Psych. service	63		Died†	2	
	Total	954	(92%)	Total	83	(8%)
IX	Study centre	818		Not seen	33	
	School or home	30		Refusals†	46	
	Psych. service	85		Died†	3	
	Overseas	22				
	Total	955	(92%)	Total	82	(8%)
XI	Study centre	803		Not seen	38	
	School or home	13		Refusals†	70	
	Psych. service	85		Died†	4	
	Overseas	24				
	Total	925	(89%)	Total	112	(11%)

*Adapted from Silva *et al.* (1984).
†Numbers of children who were refusals or who died are cumulative.

The representativeness of the sample has been largely unaffected by the loss of subjects at Phases V, VII, IX and XI. The overall distribution of the sample on the SES index has not changed significantly with the reduction in sample size. When the children assessed at 5 years were compared with those who withdrew between Phases III and V on the measures taken at Phase III, no differences were found. This was also the case for those seen and not seen at Phase VII (McGee and Silva 1982). A comparison made at Phase XI between those seen at the study centre, those seen elsewhere, those not seen because of changed location, and refusals, revealed no significant differences between any of these groups in terms of sex, IQ, reading ability, behaviour or scores on an index of disadvantage (McGee *et al.* 1984). Children of solo mothers, however, were found to be under-represented at Phase XI.

Measures

Six sets of measures were used in the study: (1) background characteristics; (2) an otological questionnaire; (3) an otological examination; (4) impedance audiometry; (5) pure-tone audiometry; (6) developmental and behavioural tests. Not all of these measures were administered at every phase of the study and there was some

TABLE 2.2
Measures administered at each phase

Measure	Phase I	III	V	VII	IX	XI
Background characteristics	√	√	√	√	√	√
Otological questionnaire	—	√	√	√	√	—
Otological examination	—	—	√	√	√	—
Impedance audiometry	—	—	√	√	√	√
Pure-tone audiometry	—	—	√	√	√	√
Developmental/behavioural	—	√	√	√	√	√

variation between phases with regard to the specific items included in each set. Table 2.2 provides an overview of the measures that were included at each phase. The specific measures are described below.

Background characteristics
Various background characteristics were recorded for the purpose of identifying risk factors associated with OME. These included information on the following: socio-economic status (SES) based on father's occupation at birth of child (Elley and Irving 1972); gestational age; weight, length and head circumference at birth, and attendance at group day-care or preschool facilities (Silva *et al.* 1981); duration of breast-feeding (Hood *et al.* 1978); history of wheezing, hay fever, eczema, bronchitis and asthma, and tests of respiratory function (Sears *et al.* 1986); and family adversity (McGee *et al.* 1984). An examination of the nose, throat and neck was made at Phases VII and IX; the month during which the child attended the study at each phase was recorded; and information on the smoking habits of parents was obtained.

Otological questionnaires
These were designed to obtain an otological history for each child. The specific questions asked at each phase are listed in Table 2.3. The three items listed for Phase III were addressed to parents during the course of a comprehensive paediatric interview and examination. At Phases V, VII and IX the questions were contained in a separate otological questionnaire administered to parents.

Otological examination
Otological examinations were conducted at Phases V, VII and IX. The items covered in each of the examinations are listed in Table 2.4. A Sparta examining microscope was used at Phase V and a Zeiss Jena microscope at Phases VII and IX. Pneumatic otoscopy was not employed.

Impedance audiometry
A Peters AP61A impedance meter with manual plot was used at Phase V and an Amplaid 704 impedance meter with Hewlett Packard XY recorder at Phases VII and IX. At Phase IX an Electromedics 86 AR automatic impedance meter (tympanometer) was used in addition to the conventional impedance meter. An evaluation of the use of the automatic impedance meter in diagnosing OME in

TABLE 2.3
Otological questionnaire items

Phase	*Item*	
III	*1.*	*Number of coughs and colds in last year.*
	2.	*Number of ear infections in last year.*
	3.	*Does your child have hearing problems?*
V	*1.*	*Do you think that . . . . . hears normally?*
	2.	*Has . . . . . ever had a real (confirmed) or suspected (not confirmed) hearing problem in the past?*
	3.	*Has . . . . . ever seen a doctor because of a suspected hearing problem?*
	4.	*Was the suspicion of a hearing problem ever confirmed?*
	5.	*Who first suspected the hearing problem?*
	6.	*At what age was the hearing problem first suspected?*
	7.	*Has . . . . . ever had any of the following problems?*
		(a) Ear infection?
		(b) Sore ears?
		(c) Pus discharge?
		If yes, what action did you take (last time)?
	8.	*Does . . . . . usually have a blocked nose?*
	9.	*How often has . . . . . had tonsillitis in the past year?*
VII	*1.*	*Do you think . . . . . ever had an accident or a near miss due to a hearing problem?*
	2.	*In the past two years has . . . . .*
		(a) had an ear infection?
		(b) been suspected of having a hearing loss?
		(c) had any ear operations? If yes, where?
IX	*1.*	*In the past two years has . . . . .*
		(a) had an ear infection?
		(b) been suspected of having a hearing loss?
		(c) had any ear operations?
	2.	*Has . . . . . had his/her tonsils out?*
		If yes, at what age?
	3.	*Has . . . . . had his/her adenoids out?*

children from another sample is reported elsewhere (Stewart *et al.* 1983). Complete agreement between automatic and conventional impedance audiometry was obtained in 89.5 per cent of cases (N = 468 ears), with the automatic impedance meter tending to produce type B curves which were not substantiated by conventional impedance audiometry. The likelihood of an artifactual type B curve is reduced if the test is repeated when a type B curve is obtained. On the basis of the above-mentioned evaluation it was decided to employ only the automatic impedance meter at Phase XI.

Tympanograms, and measures of middle-ear pressure (mmH_2O)*, pressure gradients and static compliance (expressed in terms of equivalent volume, in cm^3) were obtained from the conventional impedance audiometry conducted at Phases V, VII and IX. Tympanograms and middle-ear pressure were obtained from the automatic impedance audiometry conducted at Phases IX and XI. At Phase IX the presence or absence of an acoustic reflex was tested ipsilaterally at 1000Hz and 105dB SPL, using automatic impedance audiometry.

*Results are reported in terms of mmH_2O, the standard measure at the time the data were collected. This has since been replaced by the S.I. standard 'pascal' (Pa) unit ($9.8mmH_2O$ = 1Pa).

TABLE 2.4
Otological Examination

Phase	*Item*	
V	1.	External auditory meatus
		(a) wax
		(b) pus
		(c) crust on ear-drum
	2.	Tympanic membrane
		(a) colour
		(b) light reflex
		(c) retraction
		(d) microvascularization
		(e) calcification
		(f) scarring
		(g) thickening
		(h) adhesions
	3.	Tympanic cavity
		(a) incus necrosis
		(b) shallow attic retraction pocket
		(c) cholesteatoma
		(d) polyp or granulations
	4.	Other
VII	1.	External auditory meatus
	2.	Light reflex
	3.	Microvascularization
	4.	Calcification/hyalinization
	5.	Scarring
	6.	Translucency
	7.	Secretions
	8.	Secretion colour
	9.	Other
IX		As for Phase VII

Pure-tone audiometry

For Phase V, pure-tone thresholds at 500, 1000, 2000 and 4000Hz were measured using a Universal UAL 10 audiometer. Threshold testing at Phases VII, IX and XI was conducted using an Interacoustics AS7 audiometer with pure-tone thresholds measured as at Phase V. The audiometers were calibrated to ISO–1964 standards. Testing was conducted in a quiet but not sound-proof room.

Developmental and behavioural tests

Intelligence was assessed with the Peabody Picture Vocabulary Test (Dunn 1965) at Phase III, the Stanford–Binet Intelligence Scale (Terman and Merrill 1960) at Phase V, and the Wechsler Intelligence Scale for Children–Revised (Wechsler 1974) at Phases VII, IX and XI. Two subtests, Comprehension and Picture Arrangement, were omitted to reduce testing time and the results were prorated as recommended in the test manual.

Verbal comprehension and verbal expression were assessed at Phases III and V by the Reynell Developmental Language Scales (Reynell 1969) and at Phases VII and IX by the Auditory Reception and Verbal Expression scales of the Illinois Test of Psycholinguistic Abilities (Kirk *et al.* 1968).

Speech articulation was assessed at Phase V with the Dunedin Articulation Screening Scale (Silva 1980) and at Phases VII and IX with the Dunedin Articulation Check (Justin *et al.* 1983).

Reading was assessed at Phases VII, IX and XI with the Burt Word Reading Test (Scottish Council for Research in Education 1976).

Behaviour problems were assessed at Phases V, VII, IX and XI with the Rutter Child Scales A and B for parents and teachers respectively (Rutter *et al.* 1970; McGee *et al.* 1984).

Procedure

The paediatric interview and examination at Phase III was conducted by a paediatric physician. The otological examinations at Phases V, VII and IX were performed by a medical officer specifically trained in the use of the examining microscope. This medical officer, in an independent study on 470 ears, was found to be in 99.9 per cent agreement with the otologist involved in the present study as to the status of those ears (Stewart *et al.* 1983). The audiometrist trained for the study administered the otological questionnaire and performed the pure-tone and impedance audiometry at Phases V, VII, IX and XI. The audiometry was conducted independently of the otological examination, with the audiometrist having no knowledge of the otological findings for any child.

At Phases V, VII and IX the sequence of otological and audiological tests began with the otological examination of the child; while this was being performed the otological questionnaire was administered to the parent. Pure-tone audiometry was then performed, followed immediately by the impedance audiometry. In a few cases where testing was unsuccessful due to fatigue, the child was recalled for testing at a later date.

From Phase V, when the otological and audiological evaluations commenced, any child suspected of having an abnormality requiring further observation and/or intervention was referred to the Dunedin Hospital Otolaryngology Service. Any treatment considered clinically necessary was carried out. A small number of children had private treatment and records were available for those who did.

Missing data

As is inevitable in a study of this size, complexity and duration, it has been impossible to collect a complete set of data for every child in the sample at every phase of the study. There are many reasons for data not being collected. Of these, the most important relates to the place where the children were assessed.

The numbers of children assessed at each phase, and the various places where those assessments took place, were listed in Table 2.1. While the majority were seen at the Study Centre, several were seen at school or at home, others were seen elsewhere in the country by staff of the Department of Education's Psychological Service, and a few were seen overseas.

For those children not seen at the Study Centre, it was not possible to conduct the otological examination, impedance audiometry or pure-tone audiometry, nor was it always possible to administer the otological questionnaire or the developmental and behavioural tests. As indicated in Table 2.1, 74 children were seen away from the Study Centre at Phase V, 77 at Phase VII, 137 at Phase IX and 122 at Phase XI (the same children not necessarily being involved at each phase). These children account for the majority of the missing data acknowledged in the following chapters.

For children attending the Study Centre there were also a number of different reasons why data could not be collected, including non-cooperation or refusal to take a particular test, technical difficulties, the occasional unavailability of research staff, and time constraints imposed by the overall testing programme.

Missing data have been acknowledged throughout the following five chapters, in which the results of the study are presented, as 'missing cases', information 'not known' to the investigators, or as cases 'not examined'.

3
IDENTIFICATION AND DIAGNOSIS

In Chapter 1, five methods for identifying OME were described: history, otoscopy, impedance audiometry, pure-tone audiometry and tympanocentesis/myringotomy. The first four of these methods were used in the present study and the results of the first three are reported here. The results of the pure-tone audiometry are reported in Chapter 5.

Otological history

It was noted in Chapter 1 that the accuracy with which parents can relate the incidence of symptoms pertinent to OME is variable, especially since the disease is asymptomatic in many children. Nevertheless, otological questionnaires were administered to parents at Phases III, V, VII and IX of the study.

Phase III results

Three questions were addressed to parents at Phase III; the responses are contained in Tables 3.1 to 3.3. Of those parents responding to the questions at this phase, 92.4 per cent indicated that their child had had one or more coughs or colds in the preceding year (Table 3.1). The most frequently occurring number of coughs and colds was two, with a mean of 2.4. As indicated in Table 3.2, 26.1 per cent of the children were reported to have had one or more ear infections in the preceding year, with a mean of 0.5. Finally, 36 children (3.5 per cent) were reported to have hearing problems (Table 3.3).

Chi-square tests were conducted to determine whether there was any significant relationship between the parent reports of hearing problems and reports of coughs, colds and ear infections in the preceding year. The results are reported in Table 3.4. The first of these tests showed that there was no significant difference between the two groups with regard to coughs and colds. In contrast, a significant difference was found with regard to ear infections. Significantly more of those children with reported hearing problems had had one or more ear infections in the previous year.

Phase V results

A more detailed history was obtained from parents at Phase V. The first group of questions dealt with hearing problems and began by asking the parents if they thought their child had normal hearing. The responses to this question are presented in Table 3.5, and it is apparent that only a small number of the parents (1.7 per cent) thought that their child did not hear normally. Almost 90 per cent thought their child did hear normally, while 8.7 per cent were unsure.

Next, the parents were asked a series of questions relating to past hearing problems. The first question was intended to identify those children who had ever had a real (confirmed) or suspected (not confirmed) hearing problem in the past. For 4.8 per cent of the children, past hearing problems had been confirmed and for

TABLE 3.1

Phase III—Number of coughs and colds in the last year

Coughs/colds	*f*	%
0	75	7.6
1	215	21.9
2	299	30.4
3	202	20.5
≥4	192	19.5
	983	100.0
Not known	54	
Total sample	1037	

Mean = 2.4; standard deviation (SD) = 1.6.

TABLE 3.2

Phase III—Number of ear infections in last year

Ear infections	*f*	%
0	755	73.9
1	165	16.1
2	40	3.9
3	24	2.3
≥4	48	4.7
	1022	100.0
Not known	15	
Total sample	1037	

Mean = 0.5; SD = 1.1.

TABLE 3.3

Phase III—Does your child have hearing problems?

Response	*f*	%
No	1000	96.5
Yes	36	3.5
	1036	100.0
Not known	1	
Total sample	1037	

a further 9.5 per cent, such problems had been suspected but not confirmed (Table 3.6). For the 132 children (14.3 per cent) identified as having had past hearing problems (real or suspected), further details of these were sought from parents. The questions and the responses to them are contained in Tables 3.7 to 3.10.

Just under one-quarter (22.9 per cent) of the children with real or suspected hearing problems had never been seen by a doctor regarding these problems (Table 3.7). Most children in this group, however, had been seen by a doctor one or more times, with a mean of approximately two visits. Table 3.8 shows that for only 102 children (*i.e.* 77 per cent of the overall group) were parents able to recall whether or not a hearing problem had been confirmed. Of these children, hearing problems were confirmed in 41.

TABLE 3.4
Relationship of reported hearing problems to history of coughs, colds and ear infections at Phase III

Item	*Hearing problem* *Yes* %	*No* %	*Test statistic*
Coughs and colds	(N=32)	(N=951)	
0	3.1	7.8	
1	18.8	22.0	
2	25.0	30.6	
3	21.9	20.5	
≥4	31.3	19.1	$\chi^2(4df) = 3.70$ *ns*
Ear infections	(N=35)	(N=987)	
0	51.4	74.7	
≥1	48.6	25.3	$\chi^2(1df) = 8.29$*

*p<0.01; *ns* = not significant.

TABLE 3.5
Phase V—Do you think that your child hears normally?

Response	*f*	%
No	16	1.7
Yes	828	89.6
Unsure	80	8.7
	924	100.0
Missing cases	67	
Total sample	991	

TABLE 3.6
Phase V—Has your child ever had a real or suspected hearing problem in the past?

Response	*f*	%
No	792	85.7
Real (confirmed)	44	4.8
Suspected (not confirmed)	88	9.5
	924	100.0
Missing cases	67	
Total sample	991	

For two-thirds of the 132 children in this group, it was the mother who first suspected a hearing problem (Table 3.9). In 10 cases the problem was first suspected by staff at preschool centres attended by the children and for a further 21 children (15.9 per cent), the problem was first suspected by staff of the Dunedin study.

Table 3.10 presents the age at which hearing problems were first suspected. For 7.8 per cent of these children, this was in the first year of life, and for 6.9 per cent, in the second. A dramatic increase in the number of cases occurred in the third year of life, with 24 children (18.4 per cent) being suspected of having a hearing problem. It should be noted that the children were first seen by the

TABLE 3.7
Phase V—Has your child ever seen a doctor because of a suspected hearing problem?

Number of times	*f*	%
0	30	22.9
1	37	28.2
2	28	21.4
3	8	6.1
≥4	28	21.4
	131	100.0
Not known	1	
Total sample	132	

Mean = 2.1; SD = 2.1.

TABLE 3.8
Phase V—Was the suspicion of a hearing problem ever confirmed?

Response	*f*	%
No	61	59.8
Yes	41	40.2
	102	100.0
Not known	30	
Total	132	

TABLE 3.9
Phase V—Who first suspected the hearing problem?

Response	*f*	%
Mother	88	66.7
Father	1	0.8
Grandparent	2	1.5
Dunedin Health and Development Study	21	15.9
The Plunket Society*	5	3.8
Preschool staff	10	7.6
Other	5	3.8
Total	132	100.0

*The Plunket Society is a voluntary maternal and child health organization in New Zealand. Plunket nurses have a similar role to that of 'health visitors' in the UK.

Dunedin study at the age of 3 years and, as indicated above, 21 were suspected by the staff of the study to have hearing problems at this time. For the greatest number of children in this group (57 cases, 43.5 per cent), hearing problems were first suspected during the fourth year of life, while for the remaining 31 (23.7 per cent), such problems were first suspected in their fifth year.

A second group of questions addressed to the total sample dealt with ear infections, symptoms of ear infection, and the action taken with regard to these. The questions, and the frequency distributions of the responses to them, are

TABLE 3.10
Phase V—At what age was the problem first suspected?

Age (in months)	*f*	%
1 – 6	5	3.8
7 – 12	5	3.8
13 – 18	1	0.8
19 – 24	8	6.1
25 – 30	1	0.8
31 – 36	23	17.6
37 – 42	9	6.9
43 – 48	48	36.6
49 – 54	11	8.4
55 – 60	20	15.3
	131	100.0
Not known	1	
Total sample	132	

Mean = 41.9; SD = 13.6.

contained in Tables 3.11 to 3.16.

Table 3.11 indicates that 59.3 per cent of children had never had ear infections, 12.6 per cent had had an ear infection on one occasion, and for the remaining 28.2 per cent, ear infections had occurred on two or more occasions.

The action taken for those 376 children who had had one or more ear infections is detailed in Table 3.12. The majority (91 per cent) were seen by their family doctor and received some form of medication. 23 (6.1 per cent) were referred for specialist care and of these, 11 received surgical treatment.

As indicated in Table 3.13, 73.5 per cent of the children were believed never to have had sore ears, 10.2 per cent had had sore ears on one occasion, and the remaining 15.4 per cent had had sore ears on two or more occasions.

Of the 245 children who had had sore ears on one or more occasions, 55.6 per cent had been seen by their family doctor and 3.5 per cent had been referred to a specialist (Table 3.14). Only four children were operated on, while 53.1 per cent received medication. For a substantial proportion of these children (40.8 per cent), no action was taken by the parents.

Less than 10 per cent of the children were believed to have had a pus discharge (Table 3.15). Single episodes were reported for 4.7 per cent of the sample, and two or more episodes for 5.1 per cent. Of the 90 children with one or more episodes of pus discharge, 80 per cent were seen by their family doctor and received medication (Table 3.16). Nine children were referred to a specialist, of whom five received surgical treatment.

The final group of questions asked at Phase V was concerned with obtaining information on two disorders possibly associated with OME: blocked nose and tonsillitis. 40.7 per cent of the children were reported to have a blocked nose occasionally, 7.5 per cent frequently, and 6.0 per cent constantly, while 45.9 per cent did not usually have a blocked nose (Table 3.17).

Just over 80 per cent of the sample had not had tonsillitis in the previous year, while 11.1 per cent had had one episode and 8.7 per cent had had two or more episodes (Table 3.18).

TABLE 3.11
Phase V—Has your child ever had ear infections?

Number of times	*f*	%
0	547	59.3
1	116	12.6
2	83	9.0
3	47	5.1
≥4	130	14.1
	923	100.0
Missing cases	68	
Total sample	991	

Mean = 1.3; SD = 2.1.

TABLE 3.12
Phase V—What action did you take for your child's ear infection?

Action	*f*	%
No action	2	0.5
Saw family doctor only:		
No treatment	5	1.3
Medicine/injections	342	91.0
Saw specialist:		
Medicine	8	2.1
Other treatment	4	1.1
Operation	11	2.9
Other action	4	1.1
Total	376	100.0

TABLE 3.13
Phase V—Has your child ever had sore ears?

Number of times	*f*	%
0	678	73.5
1	94	10.2
2	79	8.6
3	26	2.8
≥4	46	5.0
	923	100.0
Missing cases	68	
Total sample	991	

Mean = 0.6; SD = 1.4.

TABLE 3.14
Phase V—What action did you take for your child's sore ears?

Action	*f*	%
No action	100	40.8
Saw family doctor only:		
No treatment	7	2.9
Medicine/injections	129	52.7
Saw specialist:		
Medicine	1	0.4
Other treatment	4	1.6
Operation	4	1.6
Total	245	100.0

TABLE 3.15
Phase V—Has your child ever had a pus discharge?

Number of times	*f*	%
0	833	90.2
1	43	4.7
2	20	2.2
3	11	1.2
≥4	16	1.7
	923	100.0
Missing cases	68	
Total sample	991	

Mean = 0.2; SD = 0.8.

TABLE 3.16
Phase V—What action did you take for your child's pus discharge?

Action	*f*	%
No action	4	4.4
Saw family doctor only:		
No treatment	2	2.2
Medicine/injections	72	80.0
Saw specialist:		
Medicine	1	1.1
Other treatment	3	3.3
operation	5	5.6
Other action	3	3.3
Total	90	100.0

TABLE 3.17
Phase V—Does your child usually have a blocked nose?

Response	*f*	%
No	424	45.9
Occasionally	376	40.7
Frequently	69	7.5
Constantly	55	6.0
	924	100.0
Missing cases	67	
Total sample	991	

TABLE 3.18
Phase V — How often has your child had tonsillitis in the past year?

Number of times	*f*	%
0	742	80.4
1	102	11.1
2	32	3.5
3	11	1.2
≥4	36	3.9
	923	100.0
Missing cases	68	
Total sample	991	

Mean = 0.4; SD = 1.2.

TABLE 3.19
Relationships of hearing problems to other disorders at Phase V

Item / *Number of episodes*	*Hearing problem* *Yes* %	*No* %	*Test statistic*
Ear infections	(N=44)	(N=879)	
0	43.2	60.1	
≥1	56.8	39.9	χ^2(1df) = 4.27*
Sore ears	(N=44)	(N=879)	
0	56.8	74.3	
≥1	43.2	25.7	χ^2(1df) = 5.69*
Pus discharge	(N=44)	(N=879)	
0	70.5	91.2	
≥1	29.5	8.8	χ^2(1df) = 18.28**
Blocked nose	(N=44)	(N=880)	
Never	52.3	45.6	
Occasionally	27.3	41.4	
Frequently	9.1	7.4	
Constantly	11.4	5.7	χ^2(3df) = 4.89 *ns*
Tonsillitis	(N=44)	(N=879)	
0	59.1	81.5	
≥1	40.9	18.5	χ^2(1df) = 11.91**

*p<0.05; **p<0.001; *ns* = not significant.

As at Phase III, the data were examined for evidence of relationships between hearing problems and other disorders. The latter included ear infections, sore ears, pus discharge, blocked nose and tonsillitis. Those children for whom hearing problems had been confirmed (Table 3.6) were compared with the remainder of the sample on each of these disorders. In each case (except for blocked nose), the sample was divided into two groups, those for whom no occurrence of the disorder had been reported, and those for whom one or more occurrences had been reported. Chi-square tests were applied and the results are reported in Table 3.19.

Significantly more of the children with confirmed hearing problems had had one or more episodes of ear infection, sore ears, pus discharge and tonsillitis than was the case for those who were reported never to have had hearing problems, the differences on the latter two variables being highly significant (p<0.001). There was no significant difference between the two groups with regard to episodes of blocked nose.

Phase VII results

At Phase VII, parents were again asked to provide a detailed otological history of their child. The first question asked whether the parents thought their child had ever had an accident or near miss due to a hearing problem. As shown in Table 3.20, 1.0 per cent considered that their child had had an accident because of a hearing problem, and a further 1.4 per cent thought their child had had a near miss for this reason.

As in previous phases of the study, parents were asked if their child had had ear infections in the past two years and, if so, on how many occasions. 39.2 per cent

TABLE 3.20
Phase VII — Do you think your child ever had an accident or a near miss due to a hearing problem?

Response	*f*	%
No	848	97.6
Yes, accident	9	1.0
Yes, near miss	12	1.4
	869	100.0
Not known	85	
Total sample	954	

TABLE 3.21
Phase VII — In the past two years has your child had any ear infection?

Response	*f*	%
No	529	60.8
Yes	341	39.2
	870	100.0
Not known	84	
Total sample	954	

TABLE 3.22
Phase VII — Number of ear infections in past two years

Number of infections	*f*	%
1	128	37.6
2	93	27.4
3	29	8.5
⩾4	90	26.5
	340	100.0
Not known	1	
Total sample	341	

Mean = 3.1; SD = 3.9.

indicated that their child had had one or more ear infections in the previous two years (Table 3.21). Of these children, 37.6 per cent had had an ear infection on only one occasion, 27.4 per cent had had infections on two occasions, 8.5 per cent on three, and the remaining 35 per cent four times or more (Table 3.22).

Parent reports of suspected hearing loss in the two years up to age 7 are presented in Table 3.23. Just over one-quarter (27.2 per cent) of the sample were suspected of having a hearing loss during this period. For 136 of these children (57.9 per cent), the hearing loss was confirmed (Table 3.24).

The number of children reported to have had ear operations in the previous two years is shown in Table 3.25. 89 children (10.3 per cent) were reported to have had ear operations, of which 18 (20.2 per cent) were for the insertion of

TABLE 3.23
Phase VII — In the past two years has your child been suspected of having a hearing loss?

Response	*f*	%
No	633	72.8
Yes	237	27.2
	870	100.0
Not known	84	
Total sample	954	

TABLE 3.24
Phase VII — Was your child's suspected hearing loss confirmed?

Response	*f*	%
No	99	42.1
Yes	136	57.9
	235	100.0
Not known	2	
Total sample	237	

TABLE 3.25
Phase VII — In the past two years has your child had any ear operations?

Response	*f*	%
No	779	89.7
Yes	89	10.3
	868	100.0
Not known	86	
Total sample	954	

TABLE 3.26
Phase VII — Ear operations

Category	*f*	%
Unilateral Tube	18	20.2
Bilateral Tubes	70	78.7
Other	1	1.1
Total	89	100.0

tympanostomy tubes unilaterally and 70 (78.7 per cent) for the insertion of tubes bilaterally (Table 3.26).

The relationship between confirmed hearing loss and parent reports of ear infections was again examined. As before, those children for whom a hearing loss had been confirmed were compared with those having normal hearing. The two groups were divided into those who had had no ear infections in the previous two years and those who had had one or more episodes of ear infection during this

TABLE 3.27
Relationship of hearing problems to ear infections at Phase VII

Number of ear infections	*Hearing problem* Yes (N=135) %	No (N=732) %	*Test statistic*
0	36.7	65.4	
≥1	63.7	34.6	χ^2(1df) = 39.43*

*p<0.001.

TABLE 3.28
Phase IX — In the past two years has your child had any ear infection?

Response	*f*	%
No	602	75.2
Yes	199	24.8
	801	100.0
Missing cases	154	
Total sample	955	

TABLE 3.29
Phase IX — How many ear infections has your child had?

Number of infections	*f*	%
1	100	50.3
2	48	24.1
3	20	10.1
≥4	31	15.6
Total	199	100.0

Mean = 2.3; SD = 2.5.

period. As Table 3.27 indicates, the two groups differed significantly, with more of those in the confirmed hearing-loss group having had one or more episodes of ear infection than was the case for those in the normal hearing group.

Phase IX results

The final otological history questionnaire was administered at Phase IX, and included the standard questions on ear infections, suspected hearing loss and ear operations. In addition, parents were asked to provide information on operations for the removal of tonsils and adenoids.

Almost one-quarter of the sample were reported to have had ear infections in the two years up to age 9 (Table 3.28). Of these 199 children, 50.3 per cent had had only one episode, 24.1 per cent had had two, 10.1 per cent had had three, and the remaining 15.6 per cent had had four or more episodes (Table 3.29).

The number of children suspected of having had hearing loss during the previous two years is reported in Table 3.30. 100 cases (12.5 per cent) were reported. In a further 15 cases hearing loss had been suspected for longer than the

TABLE 3.30
Phase IX — In the past two years has your child been suspected of having a hearing loss?

Response	*f*	%
No	686	85.6
Yes	100	12.5
Known for more than two years	15	1.9
	801	100.0
Missing cases	154	
Total sample	955	

TABLE 3.31
Phase IX — Was your child's suspected hearing loss confirmed?

Response	*f*	%
No	26	26.0
Yes	53	53.0
No attempt made to confirm	21	21.0
Total	100	100.0

TABLE 3.32
Phase IX — In the past two years has your child had any ear operations?

Response	*f*	%
No	770	95.9
Yes	33	4.1
	803	100.0
Missing cases	152	
Total sample	955	

TABLE 3.33
Phase IX — Ear operations

Category	*f*	%
Unilateral Tube	8	24.2
Bilateral Tubes	19	57.6
Other	6	18.2
Total	33	100.0

TABLE 3.34
Phase IX — Has your child had his/her tonsils out?

Response	*f*	%
No	737	91.9
Yes	65	8.1
	802	100.0
Missing cases	153	
Total sample	955	

TABLE 3.35
Phase IX — Age at which tonsils were taken out

Age (years)	*f*	%
1	9	14.3
2	29	46.0
3	1	1.6
4	2	3.2
5	8	12.7
6	4	6.3
7	6	9.5
8	1	1.6
9	3	4.8
	63	100.0
Missing cases	2	
Total sample	65	

Mean = 3.5; SD = 2.4.

TABLE 3.36
Phase IX — Has your child had his/her adenoids out?

Response	*f*	%
No	694	87.7
Yes	97	12.3
	791	100.0
Missing cases	164	
Total sample	955	

previous two years. Hearing loss had been confirmed in 53 cases, had not been confirmed in 26 cases, and in the remaining 21 cases no attempt had been made to obtain confirmation (Table 3.31).

Thirty-three children (4.1 per cent) were reported to have had ear operations in the previous two years, of whom eight (24.2 per cent) had had tympanostomy tubes inserted unilaterally and 19 (57.6 per cent) bilaterally (Tables 3.32, 3.33).

The number of children who had had their tonsils removed, and the age at which this operation was carried out, are shown in Tables 3.34 and 3.35 respectively. 65 children, or 8.1 per cent of the sample, were reported to have had their tonsils removed. For 60.3 per cent of these children, the parents stated that the operation had been conducted before the child's third birthday. To verify these parental reports, the Dunedin Hospital's records were examined (virtually all tonsillectomies in the city over this period were carried out at the Dunedin Hospital). It was found that only two children of the age-group contained in the Dunedin Study had had a tonsillectomy or adenoidectomy under the age of 3 years; neither child was included in the study group.

As reported in Table 3.36, 97 children, or 12.3 per cent of the sample, had had adenoids removed by the age of 9 years.

The relationship between confirmed hearing loss and reports of ear infections in the past two years was examined. The approach taken was the same as that

TABLE 3.37
Relationships of hearing problems to ear infections at Phase IX

Number of ear infections	*Hearing problem* Yes (N=60) %	No (N=741) %	*Test statistic*
0	38.3	78.1	
≥1	61.7	21.9	$\chi^2(1df) = 44.99$*

*p<0.001.

described for Phase VII and the results are reported in Table 3.37. Again, the groups were found to be significantly different, with more of those in the confirmed hearing-loss group having had one or more episodes of ear infection than was the case for the normal hearing group.

Summary
At each phase in which an otological history was obtained, parents were asked to report on hearing problems. Since at Phase III this question related to hearing problems at the time of the assessment, at Phase V it referred to hearing problems at any time in the past, and at Phases VII and IX to hearing problems occurring in the previous two years, it is inappropriate to compare phases. Nevertheless, it is apparent that at 3 years of age 3.5 per cent of the children were believed to have hearing problems, at 5 years 4.8 per cent had had a confirmed hearing problem sometime in the past, and at ages 7 and 9, 15.6 per cent and 6.6 per cent respectively had had a hearing loss confirmed in the previous two years. It is of interest that where parents suspected their child had a hearing problem, confirmation was obtained in 40.2 per cent of cases at age 5, 57.9 per cent at age 7 and 53.0 per cent at age 9.

At Phase V of the study, parents were questioned in detail regarding the past hearing problems of their children. Of the 924 children for whom data were available, 14.3 per cent had had a hearing problem suspected sometime in the past. Of these 132 children, 77.1 per cent had been seen by a doctor and, as noted above, 40.2 per cent had had the problem confirmed. For 66.7 per cent of these children, the problem was first suspected by their mothers and, for the majority, it was suspected in their third (18.4 per cent), fourth (43.6 per cent) or fifth (23.7 per cent) year of life.

At each phase in which the otological questionnaire was administered, a history of ear infection was obtained. At Phase III, 16.1 per cent of the children were reported to have had one or more ear infections in the preceding year. When asked at Phase V if their child had ever had an ear infection, the parents of 41.7 per cent of the children replied in the affirmative. At Phase VII, 39.2 per cent of the children had had ear infections in the preceding two years and at Phase IX, 24.8 per cent had had one or more episodes. A significant association between ear infections and hearing problems was obtained for all four phases.

At Phase V, the parents were asked if their child had ever had 'sore ears' or 'pus discharge', two symptoms of OM. The parents of 25.6 per cent of the sample indicated that their child had had sore ears on one or more occasions, while just under 10 per cent of the children were reported to have had a pus discharge on one or more occasions. Both of these symptoms were found to be significantly associated with reported hearing problems.

Also at Phase V, the parents were asked what action they had taken regarding ear infections, sore ears and pus discharge. For ear infections, 92.3 per cent of children were seen by their family doctor with 91.0 per cent receiving medication. Of the remainder, 6.1 per cent were referred for specialist care and just under half of these received surgical treatment. For two children (0.5 per cent) no action was taken. Of the 245 children who had had one or more episodes of sore ears, 55.6 per cent were seen by their family doctor and 52.7 per cent received medication. Nine children (3.6 per cent) were referred for specialist care and four (1.6 per cent) received surgical treatment. No action was taken by parents of 40.8 per cent of the children with sore ears. Of the 90 children who had had a pus discharge on one or more occasions, 82.2 per cent were seen by their family doctor and 80 per cent received medication. Nine (10.0 per cent) were referred for specialist care and five (5.6 per cent) were treated surgically. No action was taken for four (4.4 per cent) of the children with pus discharge. It is apparent from these findings that parents regarded ear infections and pus discharge more seriously than sore ears, even though all three are associated with hearing problems.

The history of a further two disorders, blocked nose and tonsillitis, was obtained at Phase V and the relationships between these and hearing problems were examined. A blocked nose was reported to have occurred occasionally for 40.7 per cent of the children, frequently for 7.5 per cent and constantly for 6.0 per cent. No relationship was found between the frequency of blocked nose and hearing problems. Just under 20 per cent of the children were reported to have had one or more episodes of tonsillitis in the year preceding their fifth birthday. A highly significant relationship between tonsillitis and hearing problems was obtained.

In Chapter 4, ear infection, sore ears, pus discharge, blocked nose and tonsillitis are examined as risk factors in the occurrence of OME.

At Phases VII and IX, the parents were asked to provide a history of ear operations in the previous two years. 89 children were reported to have had ear operations in the two years preceding their seventh birthday. Of these operations, 20.2 per cent were for the insertion of tympanostomy tubes unilaterally, and 78.7 per cent bilaterally. In the two years before their ninth birthday, 33 children had had ear operations, with 24.2 per cent of these being for the insertion of tubes unilaterally and 57.6 per cent bilaterally.

Parent reports indicated that tonsillectomies had been conducted on 63 of the children by the age of 9 years and that 60.3 per cent of these had occurred during the first two years of life. However, hospital records revealed that no tonsillectomies or adenoidectomies had been conducted on members of the cohort before the age of 3 years. This disparity must cast some doubt on the validity of the case histories, particularly with regard to chronology.

Finally, with regard to the investigation of the relationship between accidents and hearing problems, the parents of only nine children (1.0 per cent) considered that their child had had an accident due to a hearing problem, while those of a further 12 children (1.4 per cent) considered that their child had had a 'near miss' for this reason.

Otological examination

An otological examination (see Chapter 2) was conducted on each child at Phases V, VII and IX of the study. Since the examination at Phase V was the first conducted on the sample, the assessment protocol used at that time was untested and, as the following results will show, contained several items which failed to discriminate between ears with OME and ears which were normal. On the basis of the results of this first examination, a revised protocol, containing fewer items, was adopted for Phases VII and IX. In the following sections the outcome of the examination made at each phase is reported and those ears diagnosed to have OME are compared with those ears diagnosed as normal.

Outcome of the otological examination

Following the examination of each ear according to the assessment protocol, a judgement was made by the examiner as to its otological state. At Phase V, approximately 85 per cent of right and 86 per cent of left ears were judged to be normal (Table 3.38). Combining right and left ears, a total of 161 were found to contain fluid, indicating OME, while a further 22 were suspected of containing fluid. 42 ears had tympanostomy tubes present and 14 had acute otitis media, one with a perforation. Other abnormalities were detected in 13 ears (only 11 of these are recorded in the table, the remaining two ears being preferentially categorized in the foregoing groups): six ears had shallow attic retraction pockets; in a further six there was a scar adherent to the incus; and in one ear the incus tip was destroyed with adhesion of the tympanic membrane to the stapes head.

At Phase VII, approximately 89 per cent of both right and left ears were judged normal (Table 3.39). 104 ears, or approximately 6 per cent of the ears examined, were found to contain fluid, indicating OME. The examiner was uncertain as to the presence of fluid in a further 10 ears. 58 ears had tympanostomy tubes present and five had acute otitis media. Other abnormalities were detected in 17 ears, including five with perforations, five with otitis externa, three with crust obscuring the drum, two with retraction pockets, one with a haemorrhage in the tympanic membrane and one with a cholesteatoma.

At Phase IX, 94 per cent of ears were judged normal (Table 3.40). 38 ears were found to contain fluid and five were suspected of containing fluid. 15 ears had tympanostomy tubes present and one had acute otitis media. Other abnormalities were detected in 34 ears: 23 had retraction pockets; five had otitis externa; three had perforations; one was obscured by wax; one contained a foreign body; and one had had a recent myringoplasty.

Of primary interest to this study were the numbers of cases of fluid, indicating OME, identified at micro-otoscopy. Around 9 per cent of those ears examined at 5 years of age contained fluid; at 7 years this figure had declined to around 6 per cent, and at 9 years to just over 2 per cent. In contrast, the number of ears judged as normal increased from around 85 per cent at 5 years to 89 per cent at 7 years and 94 per cent at 9 years.

TABLE 3.38
Results of otological examination at Phase V

Diagnosis	*Right ear* *f*	%	*Left ear* *f*	%
Normal	729	85.0	735	85.9
Fluid definite	87	10.1	74	8.6
Fluid uncertain	12	1.4	10	1.2
Tube present in TM	20	2.3	22	2.6
Acute otitis media	4	0.5	10	1.2
Other abnormality	6	0.7	5	0.6
	858	100.0	856	100.0
Not examined	133		135	
Total sample	991		991	

TABLE 3.39
Results of otological examination at Phase VII

Diagnosis	*Right ear* *f*	%	*Left ear* *f*	%
Normal	772	88.8	775	88.9
Fluid definite	50	5.8	54	6.2
Fluid uncertain	6	0.7	4	0.5
Tube present in TM	28	3.2	30	3.4
Acute otitis media	3	0.3	2	0.2
Other abnormality	10	1.2	7	0.8
	869	100.0	872	100.0
Not examined	85		82	
Total sample	954		954	

TABLE 3.40
Results of otological examination at Phase IX

Diagnosis	*Right ear* *f*	%	*Left ear* *f*	%
Normal	761	94.5	757	93.9
Fluid definite	20	2.5	18	2.2
Fluid uncertain	2	0.2	3	0.4
Tube present in TM	7	0.9	8	1.0
Acute otitis media	0	—	1	0.1
Other abnormality	15	1.9	19	2.4
	805	100.0	806	100.0
Not examined	150		149	
Total sample	955		955	

Evidence of OME

As noted earlier, an extensive assessment protocol was employed at Phase V of the study. Percentage frequency distributions for each of the items assessed at Phase V are presented in Table 3.41, the data for right and left ears being combined for this analysis. Distributions are provided for both the 'OME' and 'Normal' groups, and the results of Chi-square tests applied to the data are reported where appropriate.

TABLE 3.41A
Otological examination at Phase V: comparison of OME and Normal groups

Item	*Diagnosis* *OME* %	*Normal* %	*Test statistic*
External auditory meatus			
(a) Wax	(N=160)	(N=1462)	
Normal	96.9	97.0	
Soft occluding meatus	2.5	2.3	
Hard occluding meatus	0.6	0.7	χ^2(2df) = 0.07 *ns*
(b) Pus	(N=161)	(N=1462)	
None/insignificant	99.4	100.0	
Yes	0.6	0.0	
(c) Crust on ear-drum	(N=160)	(N=1462)	
No	90.0	97.0	
Yes	10.0	3.0	χ^2(1df) = 17.87**
Tympanic membrane			
(a) Colour of drum	(N=160)	(N=1461)	
Normal	79.4	99.3	
Blue	5.6	0.3	
Yellow	15.0	0.4	
(b) Abnormal light reflex	(N=160)	(N=1460)	
No	21.3	81.4	
Yes	78.7	18.6	χ^2(1df) = 278.00**
(c) Retraction	(N=160)	(N=1460)	
Normal	15.0	60.5	
Very slight	45.0	30.5	
Moderate	38.8	8.6	
Extreme	1.2	0.4	χ^2(3df) = 177.58**
(d) Microvascularization	(N=160)	(N=1461)	
Grade: 0 Normal	7.5	78.8	
1 Malleus handle only	31.9	16.6	
2 } Intermediate	51.3	1.9	
3 } Intermediate	8.7	0.0	
4 Acute OM	0.6	2.7	χ^2(4df) = 774.38**

**p<0.001; *ns* = not significant.

For some items, no statistical comparison was necessary, while for others the data failed to fulfil the criteria for application of the test.

The two groups differed significantly on six of the 15 items assessed. Of those items assessed in relation to the external auditory meatus, only 'crust on ear-drum' was found to occur significantly more frequently in those ears judged to have OME. The groups did not differ in regard to wax or pus in the external auditory meatus. A crust on the ear drum, which is considered indicative of recent acute OM, was present in 10 per cent of those ears judged to have OME. In the Normal group, only 3 per cent of ears were affected in this way.

With regard to the examination of the tympanic membrane, the two groups were found to differ in the frequency with which abnormalities were observed in the colour of the drum, the light reflex, retraction of the drum, microvascularization of the drum, scarring of the drum and thickening of the membrane. The item which most clearly discriminated between the two groups was the light reflex, which was judged to be abnormal for 78.7 per cent of the OME group but only 18.6 per cent of the Normal group. While the proportions of OME cases exhibiting

TABLE 3.41B
Otological examination at Phase V: comparison of OME and Normal groups

Item	*Diagnosis*		*Test statistic*
	OME %	*Normal* %	
Tympanic membrane			
(e) Calcification	(N=160)	(N=1458)	
No	98.8	98.7	
Yes	1.2	1.3	
(f) Scar	(N=160)	(N=1460)	
No	89.4	94.1	
Atrophic	1.9	1.4	
Non-atrophic	8.7	4.5	χ^2(2df) = 5.83*
(g) Thickened	(N=160)	(N=1461)	
No	5.0	87.7	
Slight	41.9	11.6	
Definite	53.1	0.7	χ^2(2df) = 891.74**
(h) Adhesions	(N=160)	(N=1460)	
No	99.4	99.9	
Yes	0.6	0.1	
Tympanic cavity			
(a) Incus necrosis	(N=160)	(N=1462)	
No	99.4	100.0	
Yes	0.6	0.0	
(b) Shallow attic retraction pocket	(N=160)	(N=1462)	
No	98.7	99.9	
Yes	1.3	0.1	
(c) Cholesteatoma	(N=160)	(N=1462)	
No	100.0	100.0	
Yes	0.0	0.0	
(d) Polyp or granulations	(N=160)	(N=1462)	
No	100.0	100.0	
Yes	0.0	0.0	

*$p<0.05$; **$p<0.001$.

abnormal retraction of the membrane, microvascularization and thickening also clearly discriminated between the groups, the differences were not so marked for drum colour and scarring. Only 20.6 per cent of the OME group had abnormally coloured ear-drums (compared with 0.7 per cent of the Normal group) and only 10.6 per cent had scarred membranes (compared with 5.9 per cent of the Normal group). The groups did not differ with regard to calcification or adhesions.

Finally, there were no significant differences between the two groups in findings with regard to the tympanic cavity, including incus necrosis, shallow attic retraction pockets, cholesteatoma, and polyps or granulations. Very few instances of any of these signs of abnormality were observed.

As noted previously, fewer items were included in the examination protocol followed at Phase VII. Percentage frequency distributions for these items are presented in Table 3.42, as are the results of Chi-square tests applied to the data. Abnormality of the light reflex, translucency of the tympanic membrane, microvascularization, scarring, translucency and observations of secretions in the tympanic cavity were all found to discriminate between the two groups. Of the secretions observed, 75.0 per cent were neutral or grey in colour, 20.2 per cent

TABLE 3.42
Otological examination at Phase VII: comparison of OME and Normal groups

Item	*Diagnosis* *OME* %	*Normal* %	*Test statistic*
External auditory meatus	(N=104)	(N=1547)	
Normal	85.6	96.1	
Abnormal	14.4	3.9	
Light reflex	(N=104)	(N=1547)	
Normal	5.8	69.3	
Abnormal	94.2	30.7	χ^2(1df) = 170.75*
Microvascularization	(N=103)	(N=1547)	
Grade: 0 Normal	6.8	85.4	
1 Malleus handle only	36.9	14.3	
2 } Intermediate	43.7	0.3	
3 }	12.6	0.0	
4 Acute OM	0.0	0.0	χ^2(1df)† = 374.81*
Calcification/hyalinization	(N=102)	(N=1547)	
Normal	68.6	68.1	
Hyaline change	10.8	27.7	
Chalk patch	16.7	2.2	
Mixed	0.0	0.1	χ^2(1df)† = 0.0004 *ns*
Scar	(N=102)	(N=1546)	
None	86.3	94.2	
Atrophic	10.8	3.5	
Non-atrophic	2.9	2.2	
Mixed	0.0	0.1	χ^2(1df)† = 11.77*
Translucency	(N=103)	(N=1547)	
Normal	2.9	83.4	
Medial wall visible but with difficulty	22.3	13.5	
Opaque, medial wall not visible	74.8	3.1	χ^2(2df) = 739.64*
Secretions	(N=104)		
Bubbles	27.0		
With level	23.0		
Filling tympanum	50.0		
Secretion colour	(N=104)		
Neutral (grey)	75.0		
Blue	1.0		
Yellow	20.2		
White	3.8		

†Abnormal cases combined for calculation of χ^2.
*$p<0.001$; *ns* = not significant.

were yellow, 3.8 per cent were white and only one case was blue.

An almost identical pattern to that described above was obtained for the examination conducted at Phase IX. Percentage frequency distributions and Chi-square test results for this phase are presented in Table 3.43. The only notable difference in these results is that the two groups did not differ with regard to scarring of the tympanic membrane. At this phase, the examiner estimated the level of secretion visible in the tympanic cavity, whereas at Phase VII, a less precise measure had been used. For 63.2 per cent of ears in the OME group, the secretions were seen to be filling the tympanic cavity. Again, a majority of the secretions were neutral or grey in colour (64.9 per cent), while 29.7 per cent were yellow and 5.4 per cent were white. There were no cases of blue secretions.

TABLE 3.43
Otological examination at Phase IX: comparison of OME and Normal groups

Item	*Diagnosis* *OME* %	*Normal* %	*Test statistic*
External auditory meatus	(N=38)	(N=1518)	
Normal	89.5	98.4	
Abnormal	10.5	1.6	
Light reflex	(N=38)	(N=1517)	
Normal	10.5	79.1	
Abnormal	89.5	20.9	χ^2(1df) = 97.15*
Microvascularization	(N=38)	(N=1518)	
Grade: 0 Normal	10.5	91.0	
1 Malleus handle only	39.5	8.6	
2 } Intermediate	18.4	0.3	
3 }	26.3	0.1	
4 Acute OM	5.3	0.0	χ^2(1df)† = 241.51*
Calcification/hyalinization	(N=38)	(N=1516)	
Normal	65.8	65.2	
Hyaline change	21.0	28.9	
Chalk patch	13.2	3.2	
Mixed	0.0	2.7	χ^2(1df)† = 0.012 *ns*
Scar	(N=36)	(N=1518)	
None	91.7	93.9	
Atrophic	8.3	5.2	
Non-atrophic	0.0	0.9	
Mixed	0.0	0.0	χ^2(1df)† = 0.029 *ns*
Translucency	(N=38)	(N=1518)	
Normal	5.3	88.9	
Medial wall visible but with difficulty	15.8	9.8	
Opaque, medial wall not visible	78.9	1.3	χ^2(2df) = 709.39*
Secretions	(N=38)		
Bubbles	10.5		
With level	26.3		
Filling tympanum	63.2		
Secretion colour	(N=37)		
Neutral (grey)	64.9		
Blue	0.0		
Yellow	29.7		
White	5.4		

†Abnormal cases combined for calculation of χ^2.
*$p<0.001$; *ns* = not significant.

Summary

In the review of epidemiological studies in Chapter 1, it was shown that the prevalence of OME has been found to vary around a median of 13 per cent from the age of 1 year up to 6 years and then to decline rapidly to around 7 per cent at 7 years. This decline is presumed to continue beyond the age of 7 years. The results from the Dunedin study indicated slightly lower prevalence rates at the ages of 5 and 7 years, with figures of 9.4 per cent and 6.0 per cent respectively. At 9 years, the figure for this sample declined to around 2.4 per cent of those ears examined. An obvious difference between the results reported here and those reviewed in Chapter 2 is that those reported here were obtained by means of a structured otological examination using an examining microscope, while most of the epidemiological studies reviewed used the results of impedance audiometry to identify cases of OME. The present findings may therefore be considered conservative in comparison to those studies reporting impedance audiometry findings. The prevalence of OME in the present sample, based on impedance testing, is reported in Chapter 4.

The approach taken in analysing the content of the otological examination conducted at Phases V, VII and IX was to compare those ears judged by the examining otologist to have OME with those judged to be normal. From the analysis of the 15 items assessed at Phase V, it was found that only seven clearly discriminated between the two groups. Most importantly, the OME group showed an increase in abnormal light reflexes, retractions, microvascularization, scarring, thickening and abnormalities in the colour of the drum.

On the basis of the examination conducted at Phase V, a revised protocol was administered at Phases VII and IX. Of the items found redundant at Phase V, most were dropped from the subsequent examination. Since the results of the analyses of individual items at Phases VII and IX were virtually identical, only those obtained at Phase VII will be discussed. The number of ears assigned to the OME group at this age was greater than for Phase IX, thereby increasing the reliability of the analyses.

At Phase VII, the two groups were found to differ on six of the items assessed—the status of the external auditory meatus, the light reflex, microvascularization, scarring and translucency of the tympanic membrane, and secretions in the tympanic cavity.

Beyond identifying the items at Phase VII on which the groups were significantly different, the distribution of ears across levels of individual items can be examined to see which most clearly discriminate the groups. Beginning with the examination of the external auditory meatus, it can be seen that although the two groups differed on this item, only 14.4 per cent of those ears judged to have OME were assessed as abnormal in this regard. Therefore, although abnormalities of the external auditory meatus may have been observed more frequently in ears with OME, the overall occurrence of such abnormalities was relatively rare. In contrast, the second item assessed, the light reflex, was found to be abnormal in 94.2 per cent of those ears judged to have OME. Since an abnormal light reflex was observed in only 30.7 per cent of ears judged normal, this item would appear to have been a relatively reliable indicator of OME. In this context, however, it should be taken into account that an abnormal light reflex is classically considered indicative of OME; thus it may have achieved a spurious significance by conforming to the examiner's diagnosis achieved on other grounds.

Since the degree of microvascularization observed was graded on a scale of from 0 to 4, with 4 indicating acute OM, there is a need to consider the distribution of ears across these grades. As indicated in Table 3.42, whereas 93.6 per cent of ears with OME had at least some degree of microvascularization, only 14.6 per cent of normal ears were graded '1' or above. While 36.9 per cent of ears with OME were graded '1' on the above scale, compared with 14.3 per cent of normal ears, over half (56.3 per cent) of this group were graded '2' or above. This sign, therefore, also seems to have been a reliable indicator of OME.

Scarring was observed in only 14.7 per cent of ears with OME (compared with 5.7 per cent of normal ears). Therefore, as for abnormalities of the external auditory meatus, scarring of the tympanic membrane was observed in relatively few ears overall. Impaired translucency of the tympanic membrane was observed in 75.7 per cent of ears with OME but only 3.0 per cent of normal ears. This sign also appears to have been a reliable indicator of OME.

The direct observation of fluid in the tympanic cavity was, not surprisingly, the sign which most frequently and reliably discriminated cases of OME from normal ears. The colour of the secretions observed were most often judged 'neutral' (70.2 per cent), followed by 'yellow' (19.2 per cent), and 'white' (3.8 per cent).

By taking each examination item in isolation, those which most clearly discriminated abnormal (OME) from normal ears have been identified. These included an abnormal light reflex, microvascularization of the tympanic membrane, translucency of the membrane and secretions in the tympanic cavity. A diagnosis of OME would not, of course, be based on the observation of a single sign but on a combination of signs observed during examination. Observations of the appearance of the tympanic membrane cannot necessarily be regarded as objective—observer bias may result once an overall categorization has been reached either consciously or unconsciously.

Impedance audiometry

As noted in Chapter 2, a conventional impedance meter was used for the testing conducted at Phases V and VII. At Phase IX the children were tested twice, once with a conventional impedance meter and once with an automatic impedance meter. On the basis of a comparison of the results provided by the two meters both in Phase IX and with another sample (Stewart *et al.* 1983), only the automatic meter was used at Phase XI. Here the results obtained from the conventional impedance meter at Phases V, VII and IX, and from the automatic impedance meter at Phase XI are reported.

Impedance measures

In this section, the various impedance measures recorded at each phase of the study are described. These included middle-ear pressure at Phases V, VII and IX, and ipsilateral acoustic reflexes at Phases VII and IX.

MIDDLE-EAR PRESSURE

Middle-ear pressure (MEP), in mmH_2O, was obtained at four phases of the study. At Phases V, VII and IX, this was measured using conventional impedance meters, and at Phase XI, using an automatic impedance meter. Table 3.44 provides descriptive statistics for both right and left ears at each phase. MEP ranged from 0 to $-400mmH_2O$ in both ears at all phases. The test was discontinued at an MEP of $-400mmH_2O$.

Mean MEP ranged from a little over $-120mmH_2O$ in both ears at Phase V to $-84mmH_2O$ in both ears at Phase XI. A discrepancy between the means for right and left ears occurred at Phase VII. Examination of the frequency distributions at Phase VII indicated that the distribution for the left ear was more positively skewed

TABLE 3.44
Middle-ear pressure

	Phase V Right ear (N=869)	Phase V Left ear (N=859)	Phase VII Right ear (N=838)	Phase VII Left ear (N=829)	Phase IX Right ear (N=789)	Phase IX Left ear (N=780)	Phase XI Right ear (N=797)	Phase XI Left ear (N=799)
Range								
Minimum (mmH_2O)	0	0	0	0	0	0	0	0
Maximum (mmH_2O)	−400	−400	−400	−400	−400	−400	−400	−400
Mean (mmH_2O)	−126	−122	−116	−82	−89	−89	−84	−84
SD (mmH_2O)	99	99	101	89	88	90	90	90
No pressure peak† (%)	9.0	8.4	6.0	5.2	2.2	1.5	2.0	1.1
Within normal range‡ (%)	49.1	51.6	50.8	64.3	66.9	67.7	72.4	71.0

†Taken to indicate OME.
‡Normal range taken as 0 to $-100mmH_2O$.

TABLE 3.45
Static compliance

	Phase V Right ear	Phase V Left ear	Phase VII Right ear	Phase VII Left ear	Phase IX Right ear	Phase IX Left ear
Range						
Minimum (cm^3)	0.05	0.01	0.00	0.00	0.00	0.05
Maximum (cm^3)	2.75	2.55	3.30	3.40	4.00	3.20
Mean (cm^3)	0.50	0.50	0.65	0.66	0.63	0.62
SD (cm^3)	0.26	0.25	0.37	0.37	0.43	0.40
Below normal range† (%)	13.9	13.9	6.6	5.5	7.2	6.8
Within normal range (%)	85.7	85.6	90.5	91.8	89.2	89.7
Above normal range (%)	0.4	0.5	2.9	2.7	3.6	3.5

†Normal range taken as 0.3 to $1.5cm^3$.

than that for the right ear. As a consequence, when the proportion of ears falling within the normal range for MEP ($\pm 100mmH_2O$) was examined, 64.3 per cent of left ears fell into this category, compared with 50.8 per cent of right ears. While this discrepancy may have resulted in an under-representation of type C tympanograms at Phase VII (see p. 77–78), it should not have affected the detection of type B tympanograms, since these are characterized by the absence of an MEP peak. No attempt was made to adjust the data with regard to this discrepancy.

Further inspection of Table 3.44 reveals that the proportion of ears (left and right combined) with no pressure peak, indicating OME, fell from 8.7 per cent at Phase V to 1.6 per cent at Phase XI. In contrast, the proportion of ears falling within the normal range for MEP rose from 50.4 per cent at Phase V to 71.7 per cent at Phase XI.

STATIC COMPLIANCE

Static compliance was measured in terms of equivalent volume in cubic centimetres (cm^3) and data were recorded at Phases V, VII and IX of the study. Table 3.45 contains selected descriptive statistics for each ear at each of the above phases.

The mean compliance level varied little between phases and was consistent between right and left ears within phases. There was some variation both within

TABLE 3.46
Tympanometric gradient

	Phase V		*Phase VII*		*Phase IX*	
	Right ear	*Left ear*	*Right ear*	*Left ear*	*Right ear*	*Left ear*
Range						
Minimum	0.01	0.00	0.00	0.00	0.00	0.00
Maximum	0.66	0.67	0.73	0.73	0.98	0.98
Mean	0.36	0.36	0.37	0.39	0.69	0.70
SD	0.14	0.13	0.14	0.14	0.14	0.13

and between phases in the range of values recorded. Of greatest interest, however, was the number of ears at each phase which fell outside the normal limits of 0.3 to 1.5cm^3. At Phase V, 13.9 per cent of both left and right ears were below this limit, while nine ears or around 0.5 per cent exceeded it. Fewer fell below the lower limit at Phase VII, with approximately 6 per cent in this category, while just under 3 per cent exceeded the upper limit. Overall, however, a greater proportion of ears fell within the normal range, at approximately 91 per cent of those tested. At Phase IX the number of ears falling outside of normal limits rose slightly to approximately 7 per cent below 0.3cm^3 and approximately 3.5 per cent above 1.5cm^3. The increased number of ears with high compliance may indicate an increase in the number of atrophic scars following insertion of tympanostomy tubes.

TYMPANOMETRIC GRADIENT

At Phases V, VII and IX of the study, the gradients of the tympanograms produced by the impedance testing were measured. Brooks (1969) first raised the issue of defining the shape of the tympanogram and developed a measure of the gradient of the curve near its peak. This he defined as 'the change in compliance for a pressure difference of 50mm water pressure from the peak value'. Paradise and Smith (1979) redefined gradient as:

> The ratio hp/ht where ht equals the overall height of the tympanogram, and hp equals the vertical distance from the peak of the tympanogram to a horizontal line intersecting the tympanogram so its width between the points of intersection . . . is 100 mm H_2O.

Therefore, the higher this ratio, the steeper the gradient of the tympanogram. Paradise and Smith offered a procedure for classifying tympanograms, in which ears with an MEP more negative than –100mmH_2O were distinguished on the basis of gradient. They reported a higher prevalence of OME in ears with gradual gradients (<0.15) than in those with steep gradients (>0.15). Gradients measured according to Paradise and Smith's method at Phases V, VII and IX are described in Table 3.46.

There was a small increase in the range of gradients obtained between Phases V and VII. A much greater increase in the range occurred at Phase IX. Similarly, there was a very slight increase in the mean gradient between Phase V and Phase VII, but a substantial increase at Phase IX, when it rose to around 0.70. The mean gradients at all phases exceeded the value of hp/ht=0.15, which Paradise and Smith suggested as the cut-off point between gradual and steep gradients.

TABLE 3.47
Ipsilateral acoustic reflex at Phase IX (automatic meter)

*Reflex**	*Right ear*		*Left ear*	
	f	%	*f*	%
Absent	258	32.1	203	25.3
Present	545	67.9	599	74.7
	803	100.0	802	100.0
Not known	152		153	
Total sample	955		955	

*Tested at 1000Hz at 105dB SPL.

The above figures, together with an examination of the frequency distributions, suggest that a slight decline occurred between Phases V and VII in the number of tympanograms with gradual gradients, followed by an abrupt decline between Phases VII and IX. This pattern reflects the decline in the occurence of OME that would be expected at these ages.

IPSILATERAL ACOUSTIC REFLEX

Ipsilateral acoustic reflex thresholds were recorded for both ears at 1000Hz and 3000Hz at Phases VII and IX with the conventional meter. Unfortunately, these were obtained at 0mmH_2O, whereas they should have been tested at maximum compliance. This error in the testing procedure is acknowledged and, accordingly, no results are reported for this measure.

At Phase IX, the automatic impedance meter was used to test for ipsilateral acoustic reflexes at 1000Hz and 105dB SPL. The results, presented in Table 3.47, indicate that the reflex was absent in 32.1 per cent of the right ears and 25.3 per cent of the left ears tested.

Classification of ears by tympanogram type

Following collection of the impedance measures, as described above, each ear was classified on the basis of: (i) shape of the tympanogram; (ii) middle-ear pressure; (iii) static compliance. The gradient of the tympanogram was not used in this classification.

Jerger's (1970) three tympanogram types, as described in Chapter 1 (p. 18), provided the basis for the present classification. For greater precision, these were subdivided into several additional categories. The classification is described below and summarized in Table 3.48.

To allow for those cases with type A tympanograms with compliance outside the normal limits (0.3 to 1.5 cm^3), a further two categories were introduced. Those for which MEP was normal but compliance was less than 0.3cm^3—giving a 'shallow' type A tympanogram—were classified as type A_S, while those with normal MEP but with compliance exceeding 1.5cm^3—giving a 'deep' type A tympanogram —were classified as type A_D (Northern and Downs 1978).

Type C tympanograms were divided into two categories. For those ears assigned to these categories, compliance was within normal limits but MEP was

TABLE 3.48
Tympanogram types

Type	*Definition*
A	MEP peak within normal range (±100mmH_2O) and compliance within normal range (0.3 to 1.5cm^3)
A_S	MEP peak within normal range and compliance below 0.3cm^3
A_D	MEP peak within normal range and compliance above 1.5cm^3
C_1	Compliance within normal range and MEP peak within the range −101 to −200mmH_2O
C_2	Compliance within normal range and MEP peak within the range −201 to −400mmH_2O
B/C	Compliance rising as −400mmH_2O is approached but not peaking before −400mmH_2O
B	Flat or flattish curve with no measurable MEP peak
Other	Tympanogram unclassifiable

TABLE 3.49
Classification of ears by tympanogram type at each phase

Type	*Phase V*		*Phase VII*		*Phase IX*		*Phase XI*	
	Right ear	*Left ear*	*Right ear*	*Left ear*	*Right ear*	*Left ear*	*Right ear*	*Left ear*
A	404	414	403	506	493	483	471	479
A_S	23	25	15	12	19	18	71	58
A_D	—	3	6	13	15	22	37	31
C_1	184	193	196	153	147	149	116	130
C_2	165	136	156	98	89	82	79	80
B/C	15	14	4	3	7	12	10	8
B	78	74	58	43	16	12	8	12
Other	—	—	—	—	3	—	2	1
	869	859	838	828	789	778	794	799
Not known	122	132	116	126	166	177	131	126
Total	991	991	954	954	955	955	925	925

more negative than –100mmH_2O (the lower limit for normal ears). Those for which MEP fell within the range of –101 to –200mmH_2O were classified C_1, and those for which MEP fell within the range of –201 to –400mmH_2O were classified C_2.

A B/C classification was introduced for those ears which recorded a tympanogram showing compliance rising as a middle-ear pressure of –400mmH_2O was approached but not peaking before this level was reached.

A small number of tympanograms at each phase could not be assigned to any of the categories described above: these were classified as 'other'.

Table 3.49 presents the distribution of right and left ears across tympanogram types for Phases V, VII, IX and XI. The distributions for right and left ears were approximately equivalent, with the exception of Phase VII. At this phase there was a difference of just over 100 cases between right and left ears in the number of tympanograms classified as type A. A corresponding difference of just over 100 cases is apparent in the C_1 and C_2 categories. It will be recalled that when reporting the results obtained for MEP (Table 3.44), attention was drawn to an apparent discrepancy in the Phase VII data. The suggestion made at that time, that this discrepancy could result in an under-representation of type C ears, is confirmed by the present results. Since this discrepancy appeared not to significantly affect the

TABLE 3.50
Distribution of all ears by tympanogram type at each phase

Type	*Phase V*		*Phase VII*		*Phase IX*		*Phase XI*	
	f	%	*f*	%	*f*	%	*f*	%
A	818	47.3	909	54.6	976	62.3	950	59.6
A_S	48	2.8	27	1.6	37	2.4	129	8.1
A_D	3	0.2	19	1.1	37	2.4	68	4.3
C_1	377	21.8	349	21.0	296	18.8	246	15.4
C_2	301	17.4	254	15.2	171	10.9	159	10.0
B/C	29	1.7	7	0.4	19	1.2	18	1.1
B	152	8.8	101	6.1	28	1.8	20	1.3
Other	—	—	—	—	3	0.2	3	0.2
Total	1728	100.0	1666	100.0	1567	100.0	1593	100.0

remainder of the distribution, no attempt was made to adjust the data.

To simplify comparisons between phases, the distributions for right and left ears were combined to give an overall frequency for each tympanogram type at each phase. These distributions are presented in Table 3.50. They indicate a decline in the frequency of type B (including type B/C) and type C (including types C_1 and C_2) tympanograms over the four phases of the study, with a corresponding increase in the number of type A (including types A_S and A_D) tympanograms.

At Phase V, 47.3 per cent of ears were type A, indicating normal MEP and compliance. Of the 39.2 per cent of ears with type C tympanograms, 21.8 per cent were classified C_1 and 17.4 per cent C_2. Only a small number of ears (1.7 per cent) were assigned to the B/C category. Finally, 8.8 per cent of ears had type B tympanograms, indicating OME.

Phase VII saw a slight decline in the frequency of abnormal tympanograms, with a corresponding increase in tympanometrically normal ears. Almost 55 per cent of tympanograms were type A at this phase, while the number of type B tympanograms declined to 6.1 per cent of those tested. There was a similar decline in the frequency of ears with MEP more negative than $-100mmH_2O$.

A more abrupt decline in abnormal tympanograms can be seen at Phase IX, with type B dropping to 1.8 per cent, type C_1 to 18.8 per cent, and type C_2 to 10.9 per cent. Tympanometrically normal ears (type A) increased to 62.3 per cent at this phase.

At Phase XI, the proportion of type B tympanograms had declined to 1.3 per cent, of type C_1 to 15.4 per cent and of type C_2 to 10 per cent. The increases in type A_S to 8.1 per cent and in type A_D to 4.3 per cent indicate increased tympanic membrane pathology, albeit minor, presumably a result of OME or its treatment.

Since the prevalence rates for differing tympanogram types in the sample are fully reported in Chapter 5, the above results are not examined further here.

Summary

Middle-ear pressure was found to range from 0 to -400 mmH_2O at all four phases, with a mean of around $-120mmH_2O$ at Phase V, declining to $-84mmH_2O$ at Phase XI. The proportion of ears with no pressure peak fell from 8.7 per cent at Phase V to 1.6 per cent at Phase XI.

Static compliance was recorded at Phases V, VII, and IX of the study, and it was found that the majority of ears fell within the normal limits of 0.3 to 1.5cm^3. Ears with compliance lower than 0.3cm^3 declined from 14 per cent at Phase V to 7 per cent at Phase IX. Ears with compliance higher than 1.5cm^3 increased from 0.5 per cent at Phase V to 3.5 per cent at Phase IX.

The gradients of the tympanograms obtained at Phases V, VII and IX were calculated according to the method of Paradise and Smith (1979). The range of gradients obtained at Phase V (0 to 0.67) and at Phase VII (0 to 0.73) were lower than those recorded at Phase IX (0 to 0.98). The mean gradients also were lower at Phases V (around 0.67) and VII (0.73) than at Phase IX (0.98).

Ipsilateral acoustic reflex testing conducted with an automatic impedance meter at Phase IX indicated that reflexes were absent in 32.1 per cent of right ears and 23.5 per cent of left ears.

Each ear tested at each phase was classified by tympanogram type, based on the shape of the tympanogram obtained for that ear, its MEP, and its static compliance. The results reported above indicated that a slight decline in type B and type C (C_1 and C_2) ears occurred between Phases V and VII, with a more abrupt decline occurring between Phases VII and IX. There was a further slight decline in these types between Phases IX and XI. A small and declining number of ears were assigned to the B/C category over the four phases of the study. Corresponding increases in type A (A, A_S and A_D) ears occurred over the four phases. Of greatest interest was the decline in type B ears from 8.8 per cent at Phase V to 6.1 per cent at Phase VII, 1.8 per cent at Phase IX, and 1.3 per cent at Phase XI. It is notable that these figures are consistent with those obtained from the otological examination reported earlier. Type C ears declined from 39.2 per cent at Phase V to 25.4 per cent at Phase XI. Type B/C ears declined from 1.7 per cent at Phase V to 1.1 per cent at Phase XI. Type A ears increased from 50.3 per cent at Phase V to 72.0 per cent at Phase XI.

No further analyses were conducted on the data reported in this section, since its primary pupose was to report the results of the impedance audiometry conducted at each phase and to describe the classification of ears by tympanogram type. This classification provided the basis for grouping subjects in subsequent analyses, reported in Chapters 4 ('Epidemiology and risk factors.'), 5 ('Audiological characteristics.') and 6 ('Developmental consequences').

Comparison of impedance audiometry and otological examination

In this chapter, findings on three methods of detection of OME—history, otological examination and impedance audiometry—have been reported. Since the otological examination and impedance audiometry were the principal methods of detection used in this study, it is appropriate that the correspondence between them be examined here. The otological history, on the other hand, being concerned with reports of past episodes of hearing problems, ear infections and related disorders, is not included in this comparison. The examination of risk factors asociated with OME is dealt with in Chapter 4.

One difficulty in comparing the findings of the impedance audiometry with those of the otological examination is the difference in levels of categorization

TABLE 3.51
Examination decision by tympanogram type at Phase V

Type		*Otological diagnosis*								*Total*
		Normal		*Fluid*		*Uncertain*		*Other*		
		f	%	*f*	%	*f*	%	*f*	%	
A		757	98.7	3	0.4	4	0.5	3	0.4	767
	%	53.0		1.9		18.2		12.5		
A_S		41	93.2	1	2.3	2	4.5	—	—	44
	%	2.9		0.6		9.1		—		
A_D		3	100.0	—	—	—	—	—	—	3
	%	0.2		—		—		—		
C_1		342	94.8	7	1.9	3	0.8	9	2.5	361
	%	24.0		4.4		13.7		37.5		
C_2		250	88.3	26	9.2	5	1.8	2	0.7	283
	%	17.5		16.3		22.7		8.3		
B/C		11	37.9	16	55.3	1	3.4	1	3.4	29
	%	0.8		10.0		4.5		4.2		
B		23	15.7	107	73.3	7	4.8	9	5.2	146
	%	1.6		67.0		31.8		37.5		
Total		1472		160		22		24		1633

TABLE 3.52
Examination decision by tympanogram type at Phase VII

Type		*Otological diagnosis*								*Total*
		Normal		*Fluid*		*Uncertain*		*Other*		
		f	%	*f*	%	*f*	%	*f*	%	
A		894	99.3	2	0.2	1	0.1	4	0.4	901
	%	58.9		2.0		12.5		19.0		
A_S		24	88.9	1	3.7	2	7.4	—	—	27
	%	1.6		1.0		25.0		—		
A_D		17	94.4	—	—	—	—	1	5.6	18
	%	1.1		—		—		4.8		
C_1		331	95.9	8	2.3	1	0.3	5	1.5	345
	%	21.8		7.8		12.5		23.8		
C_2		228	90.1	22	8.7	1	0.4	2	0.8	253
	%	15.0		21.6		12.5		9.5		
B/C		6	85.7	1	14.3	—	—	—	—	7
	%	0.4		1.0		—		—		
B		18	18.4	68	69.4	3	3.0	9	9.2	98
	%	1.2		66.6		37.5		42.9		
Total		1518		102		8		21		1649

associated with each. Whereas the examiner assigned ears to one of four broad categories—normal, fluid, uncertain, and other abnormalities including the presence of tubes and acute OM—the impedance audiometry produced a more complex classification, with seven categories based on three dimensions: shape of the tympanogram, middle-ear pressure and static compliance. Accordingly, ears with no indication of fluid on examination may, nevertheless, have had abnormal MEP or compliance when tested with the impedance meter. To assess the degree of correspondence between these two methods of identification, the two sets of results were cross-tabulated. The results of these cross-tabulations are displayed in Tables 3.51 (Phase V), 3.52 (Phase VII) and 3.53 (Phase IX). It should be noted that a

TABLE 3.53
Examination decision by tympanogram type at Phase IX

Type		*Otological diagnosis*								*Total*
		Normal		*Fluid*		*Uncertain*		*Other*		
		f	%	*f*	%	*f*	%	*f*	%	
A		953	99.3	2	0.2	—	—	5	0.6	960
	%	65.0		5.7		—		14.3		
A_S		36	100.0	—	—	—	—	—	—	36
	%	2.4		—		—		—		
A_D		33	91.7	—	—	—	—	3	8.3	36
	%	2.3		—		—		8.6		
C_1		278	95.2	4	1.4	2	0.7	8	2.7	292
	%	19.0		11.4		40.0		22.8		
C_2		147	88.0	8	4.8	2	1.2	10	6.0	167
	%	10.0		22.9		40.0		28.6		
B/C		12	63.2	2	10.5	1	5.3	4	21.0	19
	%	0.8		5.7		20.0		11.4		
B		6	21.4	18	64.3	—	—	4	14.3	28
	%	0.4		51.4		—		11.4		
Other		1	33.3	1	33.3	—	—	1	33.4	3
	%	0.1		2.9		—		2.9		
Total		1466		35		5		35		1541

number of cases have been lost to this analysis due to the unavailability of data for certain of the measures. Also, since for the majority of tube cases no tympanogram was recorded, all tube cases were excluded from this analysis.

To assist in the interpretation of these results, each frequency has been expressed in the tables both as a proportion of the total number of cases in each column (percentage below the frequency figure) and as a proportion of the total number of cases in each row (percentage alongside the frequency figure). The percentages below the frequency figures in each column, therefore, represent the number of cases under that category of otological diagnosis which were assigned to each of the seven tympanogram types. Similarly, the percentages alongside the frequency figures in each row represent the number of cases with that tympanogram type which were assigned to each category of otological diagnosis.

Table 3.51 shows that of the 1427 cases categorized as normal by the examiner, only 757 (53 per cent) had type A tympanograms. Of the remaining ears judged to be normal, the great majority had type C_1 (24 per cent) or type C_2 (17.5 per cent) tympanograms.

Of the 160 ears found to have fluid present on examination, 107 (67 per cent) had a type B tympanogram. 10 per cent were type B/C and almost 21 per cent were type C. Where the examiner was uncertain as to the presence of fluid, 31.8 per cent of ears were found to have type B tympanograms, 4.5 per cent type B/C, and 36.4 per cent type C. 27 per cent of the ears in this category had type A tympanograms.

Comparing the otological examination findings with tympanogram types, it was found that of the 767 ears with type A tympanograms, 98.7 per cent were considered normal on examination. Similarly high percentages of those with type A_S (93.2 per cent), A_D (100 per cent), and C_1 (94.8 per cent) tympanograms were judged normal on examination. A slightly lower proportion of ears with type C_2

TABLE 3.54
Microscopically diagnosed effusion by tymPanogram type at Phase VII

Effusion	*Type A*		*Type B*		*Type C_1*		*Type C_2*		*Total*
	f	%	*f*	%	*f*	%	*f*	%	
None	941	61.1	32	2.1	337	21.9	229	14.9	1539
Partially filling tympanum	1	1.9	31	58.5	7	13.2	14	26.4	53
Filling tympanum	2	3.8	40	76.9	1	1.9	9	17.3	52

tympanograms were judged normal (88.3 per cent), with 9.2 per cent being found to have fluid on examination. Of those with type B tympanograms, 73.3 per cent were judged to have fluid present on examination and 15.7 per cent were judged normal, while for 4.8 per cent the examiner was uncertain as to the presence of fluid. Finally, of those ears with type B/C tympanograms. 55.3 per cent were judged to have fluid present and in a further 3.4 per cent there was uncertainty as to the presence of fluid. 11 B/C type ears (37.9 per cent) were judged normal on examination.

The cross-tabulations for Phases VII and IX were generally similar to those just described. One notable difference was in the otological diagnoses made for those ears with type B/C tympanograms. At Phase V, 55.3 per cent were judged to have fluid and 37.9 per cent were judged to be normal. In contrast, at Phase VII, 14.3 per cent were judged to have fluid and 85.7 per cent were judged normal. Similar figures were obtained at Phase IX.

Secretions

Given the above findings it was of interest to examine the relationship between secretions observed at examination and the tympanogram types to which ears were assigned. Since information on secretions was first recorded at Phase VII, the above relationship was examined using the data from this phase. Tympanogram types were categorized according to the examiner's decision as to whether the middle-ear cavity was clear of secretion, partially filled with secretion or completely filled with secretion. The results of this categorization are shown in Table 3.54.

The typical finding with a middle-ear effusion was a type B tympanogram (67.6 per cent of all cases). A proportion of middle-ear effusions were associated with type C tympanograms (29.5 per cent), particularly type C_2 (21.9 per cent). Where a type C_1 tympanogram was associated with middle-ear effusion, it was most likely that the secretions only partially filled the tympanic cavity. In only three of the 941 type A ears did the examiner observe secretions in the tympanic cavity.

Discussion

Several observations can now be made regarding the degree of correspondence between the two main methods of identification of OME, otological examination and impedance audiometry. Since the results obtained at Phases V, VII and IX were generally similar, this discussion is based on those for Phase V only.

The data obtained at Phase V confirmed the earlier expectation that ears judged ‘normal’ on examination may be found to have abnormal MEP or compliance when tested with an impedance meter. This was found to be the case for 47 per cent of ears judged normal at Phase V. The broad categorization used by the examiner in this study, being based on observations of structure rather than functioning, did not allow for the identification of functional abnormalities such as abnormal MEP or low compliance.

With regard to the identification of OME, there was agreement between the two methods in 107 cases, or 54 per cent of the total number of OME cases identified by the two methods. Of the 160 cases identified by the examiner, only 107 (67 per cent) had type B tympanograms. Conversely, of the 146 cases with type B tympanograms, only 73 per cent were judged by the examiner to have OME.

Little can be said about the ability of impedance audiometry to resolve uncertainty with regard to the presence of fluid in the tympanic cavity. At Phase V, less than one-third of such cases were found to have type B tympanograms and only 18 per cent had type A tympanograms. The majority of the remaining cases were found to have middle-ear pressure more negative than $-100mmH_2O$.

Of the 767 ears found to have type A tympanograms at Phase V, 98.7 per cent were judged normal by the examiner, indicating a high level of agreement between the two methods in this regard.

When the relationship between secretions observed at examination and tympanogram types was investigated, it was clearly shown that the typical finding with a midddle-ear effusion was a type B tympanogram.

4
EPIDEMIOLOGY AND RISK FACTORS

Recent research on the epidemiology of OME and on risk factors associated with this disease were reviewed in Chapter 1. Several deficiencies in the literature were identified, including the paucity of data on the epidemiology of the disease in children over the age of 7 years, and particularly in New Zealand children. It was noted that existing knowledge regarding many of the risk factors was equivocal. The present chapter will address these issues.

Prevalence

It was noted in Chapter 1 that the criterion most often used in recent epidemiological studies to identify cases of OME was the type B tympanogram. In order to compare the present study with earlier reports, the same criterion was adopted for the analyses reported below. Similarly, to enable comparison with the majority of the studies reviewed in Chapter 1, the prevalence rates reported below are for 'ears'. Later in this section rates for 'children' are reported.

The classification of the present sample by tympanogram type has already been fully reported in Chapter 3. Seven tympanogram types were defined. Here the seven types have been grouped into three major categories: Type A (including types A_S and A_D); Type B (including type B/C); and Type C (including types C_1 and C_2).

Table 4.1 presents the distribution of the sample across these categories at Phases V, VII, IX and XI of the study. Separate distributions for right and left ears have been provided. In those cases where a tympanogram could not be classified, the ear concerned was assigned to a category labelled 'other'. For the purpose of calculating prevalence rates, the distributions for right and left ears were combined.

The combined distributions are presented in Table 4.2. The prevalence of type B tympanograms at the age of 5 years is shown to be 10.5 per cent. This is likely to provide an underestimate of ears with OME, for reasons described in the previous chapter. On the other hand, ears showing B tympanograms at the age of 5 years are likely to have significant OME. The prevalence declined to 6.5 per cent at 7 years, 3.0 per cent at 9 years and 2.4 per cent at 11 years. The prevalence of type C tympanograms in ears at 5 years was 39.2 per cent, declining to 36.2 per cent at 7 years, 29.8 per cent at 9 years and 25.4 per cent at 11 years. The prevalence of type A tympanograms in ears increased steadily, from 50.3 per cent at age 5 to 72.0 per cent at age 11.

Since it was of interest to know how many children in the sample had the differing tympanogram types at each phase of the study, each child was assigned to one of five categories, according to the status of his or her two ears: (i) Bilateral A; (ii) Bilateral B; (iii) Unilateral B; (iv) Bilateral C; (v) Unilateral C. In the case of the Unilateral B and Unilateral C categories, the contralateral ear was disregarded. The distribution of the sample across these categories at each phase is recorded in Table 4.3.

TABLE 4.1
Distribution of right and left ears by tympanogram type at each phase

Type	*Phase V*		*Phase VII*		*Phase IX*		*Phase XI*	
	Right	*Left*	*Right*	*Left*	*Right*	*Left*	*Right*	*Left*
A	427	442	424	531	527	523	579	568
B	93	88	62	46	23	24	18	20
C	349	329	352	251	236	231	195	210
Other	—	—	—	—	3	—	2	1
	869	859	838	828	789	778	794	799
Missing	122	132	116	126	166	177	131	126
Total	991	991	954	954	955	955	925	925

TABLE 4.2
Distribution of all ears by tympanogram type at each phase

Type	*Phase V*		*Phase VII*		*Phase IX*		*Phase XI*	
	f	%	*f*	%	*f*	%	*f*	%
A	869	50.3	955	57.3	1050	67.0	1147	72.0
B	181	10.5	108	6.5	47	3.0	38	2.4
C	678	39.2	603	36.2	467	29.8	405	25.4
Other	—	—	—	—	3	0.2	3	0.2
Total	1728	100.0	1666	100.0	1567	100.0	1593	100.0

TABLE 4.3
Distribution of children by tympanogram type of both ears at each phase

Group	*Phase V*		*Phase VII*		*Phase IX*		*Phase XI*	
	f	%	*f*	%	*f*	%	*f*	%
Bilateral A	347	40.5	369	45.0	439	57.1	499	63.2
Bilateral B	51	6.0	24	2.9	12	1.6	10	1.3
Unilateral B	78	9.1	54	6.6	21	2.7	17	2.2
Bilateral C	232	27.0	188	22.9	145	18.9	126	15.9
Unilateral C	149	17.4	185	22.6	151	19.7	138	17.5
Total	857	100.0	820	100.0	768	100.0	790	100.0

At 5 years of age, 15.1 per cent of the children tested were found to have type B tympanograms either bilaterally or unilaterally. This figure declined to 9.5 per cent at 7 years, 4.3 per cent at 9 years and 3.5 per cent at 11 years. This final figure was obtained despite the fact that only the automatic impedance meter, which tends to overdiagnose type B tympanograms, was used at Phase XI. Additionally, calcification of the drum may produce a type B tympanogram and is more likely to have developed at this age, again providing an overestimate of OME if defined by a B tympanogram. It is clear from Table 4.3 that there were more cases of unilateral B tympanograms than bilateral B tympanograms at each phase. The ratio of unilateral to bilateral cases was approximately 1.5:1 at Phase V, 2:1 at Phase VII, and 1.7:1 at both Phase IX and Phase XI.

A relatively large proportion of the sample was found to register type C tympanograms in one or both ears at the time of testing. At age 5, 44.4 per cent of the children were assigned to either the Bilateral C or Unilateral C groups. At age 7, 45.5 per cent were assigned to these groups. Thereafter the prevalence declined, to 38.6 per cent at 9 years and 33.4 per cent at 11 years. The proportions of children with bilateral and unilateral type C tympanograms were approximately equal at Phases VII, IX and XI, while at Phase V the proportion in the Bilateral C group was higher by aproximately 10 per cent.

In contrast to the above, the proportion of the sample with two normal tympanograms (Bilateral A) increased steadily, from 40.5 per cent at Phase V to 45 per cent at Phase VII, 57.1 per cent at Phase IX and 63.2 per cent at Phase XI.

Tympanostomy tubes

A factor not taken into account when calculating the prevalence rates reported above was the number of ears which had tympanostomy tubes in place at the time of testing. From the findings of the otological examination conducted at Phases V, VII and IX, it was possible to identify the cases concerned and to assign these ears to a 'tubes' category at each phase. The resulting prevalence rates for ears are presented in Table 4.4. It should be noted that tympanograms were recorded for some ears which had tympanostomy tubes in place and that these cases were included in the distributions of tympanogram types reported in Table 4.1 (and associated tables). For the distributions presented in Table 4.4 these ears were reassigned to the 'tubes' category. Accordingly, in Table 4.4 (and associated tables) some of the tympanogram categories at each phase contain fewer cases than the corresponding categories in Table 4.1 (and associated tables).

As before, the distributions for the two ears were combined and these are presented in Table 4.5. It can be seen that 2.6 per cent of ears had tubes in place at Phase V, 3.4 per cent at Phase VII and 0.9 per cent at Phase IX. Since no otological examination was conducted at Phase XI, no record of tubes in place was available for this phase.

The presence of tympanostomy tubes prevents an accurate estimate of the prevalence of OME. It does seem reasonable from an epidemiological viewpoint, however, to combine ears with tympanostomy tubes with those showing B tympanograms, as tympanostomy tubes in general remain in the ear for a limited period. This will give a slight overestimate of prevalence (some effusions may have resolved spontaneously over the period when the tubes were in) but appears legitimate, as excluding this group would almost certainly provide a relatively greater underestimate. It is pertinent to recall that Tos *et al.* (1983*b*), in their study of OME in preschool children, likewise assigned ears with open tympanostomy tubes to the type B category.

From Table 4.5 it can be seen that the 'combined' prevalence rates at ages 5, 7, 9 and 11 years were 12.5, 9.4, 3.5 and 2.4 per cent respectively. The prevalence rates for the other groups were largely unaffected by this reassignment of cases.

Again, it was of interest to know how many children had type B tympanograms, had tubes inserted, or had middle-ear pressure more negative than $-100mmH_2O$. Each child was assigned to one of the following seven groups: (i) Bilateral A; (ii) Bilateral B; (iii) Unilateral B; (iv) Bilateral Tubes; (v) Unilateral Tube; (vi) Bilateral C; (vii) Unilateral C. In the case of the Unilateral B, Uni-

TABLE 4.4
Status of right and left ears at each phase

Status	*Phase V*		*Phase VII*		*Phase IX*		*Phase XI*	
	Right	*Left*	*Right*	*Left*	*Right*	*Left*	*Right*	*Left*
Type A	427	442	424	530	524	522	579	568
Type B	91	85	57	45	21	20	18	20
Tubes	21	25	28	30	7	8	—	—
Type C	348	329	348	248	236	228	195	210
Other	—	—	—	—	3	—	2	1
Total	887	881	857	853	791	778	794	799

TABLE 4.5
Status of all ears at each phase

Status	*Phase V*		*Phase VII*		*Phase IX*		*Phase XI*	
	f	%	*f*	%	*f*	%	*f*	%
Type A	869	49.2	954	55.8	1046	66.7	1147	72.0
Type B	176	9.9	102	6.0	41	2.6	38	2.4
Tubes	46	2.6	58	3.4	15	0.9	—	—
Type C	667	38.3	596	34.8	464	29.6	405	25.4
Other	—	—	—	—	3	0.2	3	0.2
Total	1768	100.0	1710	100.0	1569	100.0	1593	100.0

TABLE 4.6
Distribution of children by the status of both ears at each phase

Group	*Phase V*		*Phase VII*		*Phase IX*		*Phase XI*	
	f	%	*f*	%	*f*	%	*f*	%
Bilateral A	347	39.4	369	43.6	436	56.6	499	63.2
Bilateral B	49	5.6	24	2.8	8	1.0	10	1.3
Unilateral B	78	8.8	50	5.9	19	2.5	17	2.2
Bilateral Tubes	20	2.3	20	2.4	2	0.3	—	—
Unilateral Tube	6	0.7	15	1.8	11	1.4	—	—
Bilateral C	232	26.3	184	21.7	144	18.7	126	15.9
Unilateral C	149	16.9	185	21.8	150	19.5	138	17.5
Total	881		847		770		790	

lateral C and Unilateral Tube groups, the contralateral ear was disregarded. The distribution of the sample across these seven groups, at each phase, is indicated in Table 4.6.

Combining the two B groups and the two Tube groups gives an estimate of how many children were likely to be affected by OME in one or both ears at the time of testing at each phase of the study. At 5 years of age, 17.4 per cent of the sample were found to be affected, declining to 12.9 per cent at 7 years, 5.2 per cent at 9 years, and 3.5 per cent at 11 years.

Discussion
In the above sections, the prevalence of OME in the sample at the ages of 5, 7, 9 and 11 years is estimated. Using a type B tympanogram as evidence of OME, prevalence rates for *ears* of 10.5 per cent and 6.5 per cent at ages 5 and 7 years

respectively were obtained. These rates are comparable to those reported in the studies reviewed in Chapter 1.

In the study reported by Tos *et al.* (1983*b*), ears with tympanostomy tubes in place were included with those with type B tympanograms to give the prevalence rates reported. In the present study, when those children with tympanostomy tubes present at the time of testing were included in the calculation of the prevalence rates, these increased to 12.5 per cent at 5 years and 9.4 per cent at 7 years. Rates both with and without tube cases have been included here in order to give a comprehensive description of the prevalence of OME in the Dunedin sample.

As noted in Chapter 1, prevalence rates for *children* over the age of 7 years have not been reported elsewhere in the literature, although it is recognized clinically that the prevalence of OME declines quite rapidly from the age of 6 years on. The Dunedin data support this view: at 5 years the rate was 15.1 per cent, decreasing to 9.5 per cent at 7 years, 4.3 per cent at 9 years and 3.5 per cent at 11 years. Of the children involved, however, fewer were affected bilaterally than were affected unilaterally at any age. The prevalence rates for children with bilateral B tympanograms were 6.0 per cent at 5 years, 2.9 per cent at 7 years, 1.6 per cent at 9 years, and 1.3 per cent at 11 years. These figures suggest that only a comparatively small proportion of children in the age-groups reported in this study are affected bilaterally by OME.

When the children with tubes in place at the time of testing were included in the prevalence figures, these rose to 17.4 per cent at 5 years, 12.9 per cent at 7 years, 5.2 per cent at 9 years and 3.5 per cent at 11 years. Whereas the ratio of unilateral to bilateral OME cases ranged from 1.5:1 to 2:1, a higher proportion of children had tubes bilaterally than had them unilaterally. At 5 years of age, 20 children had tubes bilaterally, compared with only six unilaterally. At 7 years of age, 20 children had tubes bilaterally and 15 had them unilaterally. These figures reflect local treatment strategies.

When the findings for tympanometrically normal ears were examined (Table 4.2), it was clear that the proportion of these in the sample had risen steadily with age. At 5 years, 50.3 per cent of ears were in this group; by 11 years this figure had increased to 72.0 per cent. Similarly, when the children with both ears normal at each age were considered (Table 4.3), the figure was seen to rise from 40.5 per cent at 5 years to 63.2 per cent at 11 years. In spite of this steady improvement over the years, it was clear that even at 11 years of age a substantial proportion of the sample fell outside a strictly defined tympanometric norm, with 28.0 per cent of ears and 36.8 per cent of children in this group. The main contribution to these figures was made by type C rather than type B tympanograms. As noted earlier, a relatively high proportion of the sample at each age had type C tympanograms when tested. The contribution made by the type C group to the total number of abnormal tympanograms increased with age, while that made by the type B group declined. At 5 years of age, 79 per cent of ears with abnormal tympanograms were in the type C group; by 11 years this figure had increased to 91 per cent. The type C tympanogram is ubiquitous in childhood and it may well be that a different norm of middle-ear pressure than that defined for the adult population (Jerger 1970) is appropriate in childhood.

TABLE 4.7
Groups used in the investigation of risk factors

Group	*Definition*	*N*
1	Persistent* bilateral OME, with or without tympanostomy tubes	98
2	Persistent* unilateral OME, with or without tympanostomy tubes	26
3	Transient** unilateral or bilateral OME	118
4	Never proven OME, scarred tympanic membrane	138
5	Ears showing a type C tympanogram on at least one occasion but never OME or a type B tympanogram	449
6	Never proven OME, no scarred tympanic membranes, always bilateral A tympanogram when assessed	133
Total sample		962

**Persistent.* The effusion was observed at the Study Centre or Department of Otolaryngology to last for a three month period or longer. In general the criteria for inserting tympanostomy tubes included a duration of effusion of three months or longer.
***Transient.* One or at most two episodes of middle-ear effusion were recorded on attendance at the Study Centre or Department of Otolaryngology but these episodes were of less than three months duration, often considerably less.

Incidence and natural history

What little information has been published on the incidence of OME was reviewed in Chapter 1. Because of the design of the present study it was not possible to contribute any findings in this area. From what is known of the natural history of OME, and given that the present sample was tested only once every two years, it would be inappropriate to report incidence rates. Similarly, this study was not designed to contribute information on the natural history of OME.

Risk factors

In this section an investigation of several factors which have possible aetiological significance for OME is reported. The review of literature on this subject indicated that the evidence on many factors was equivocal and that further research was required. While not all of the factors considered in Chapter 1 were included in the present investigation, many were, and the findings on each of these are related back to the earlier evidence. The order in which the various risk factors are examined here follows that used in Chapter 1. As before, they are divided into 'host' and 'environmental' factors.

For the purpose of this investigation the sample was divided into six longitudinal groups based on the study data and records of the Dunedin Hospital Otolaryngology Service, up to the age of 9 years. The six groups are defined in Table 4.7 and the number of children assigned to each group is given. Data on a total of 962 children were available for this analysis. For the investigation of some risk factors, the above groupings were inappropriate and where this was the case the groupings used are described in the text.

Host factors

Age, sex, socio-economic status, infant nutrition, related disorders and perinatal characteristics were investigated and the results are reported in the following sections. Statistical test results for the majority of these factors are presented in Table 4.8.

TABLE 4.8
Results from the investigation of host factors

Risk factor	*Test statistic*	
Sex	$\chi^2(5df) = 12.25$	*
Socio-economic status	$\chi^2(10df) = 13.73$	*ns*
Breastfeeding	$\chi^2(10df) = 30.35$	***
History of ear infection		
Phase V	$\chi^2(10df) = 31.06$	***
Phase VII	$\chi^2(10df) = 86.29$	***
History of sore ears	$\chi^2(5df) = 32.04$	***
History of purulent ear discharge		
Phase V	$\chi^2(5df) = 64.91$	***
Phase VII	$\chi^2(5df) = 8.74$	*ns*
History of nasal obstruction	$\chi^2(10df) = 27.63$	**
Clinical diagnosis of nasal obstruction	$\chi^2(10df) = 20.54$	*
Turbinate size	$\chi^2(5df) = 4.92$	*ns*
History of tonsillitis	$\chi^2(5df) = 14.41$	*
Tonsil size	$\chi^2(15df) = 19.25$	*ns*
Cervical adenitis	$\chi^2(10df) = 12.44$	*ns*
History of wheezing	$\chi^2(15df) = 15.99$	*ns*
History of hay fever	$\chi^2(5df) = 0.91$	*ns*
History of eczema	$\chi^2(5df) = 2.71$	*ns*
History of bronchitis	$\chi^2(5df) = 3.33$	*ns*
History of asthma	$\chi^2(10df) = 3.56$	*ns*
Hyper-reactive airways	$\chi^2(15df) = 6.58$	*ns*
Gestational age	$F(5, 843df) = 0.22$	*ns*
Birthweight	$F(5, 956df) = 1.09$	*ns*
Length at birth	$F(5, 954df) = 0.70$	*ns*
Head circumference at birth	$F(5, 956df) = 0.66$	*ns*

*$p<0.05$; **$p<0.01$; ***$p<0.001$; *ns* = not significant.

AGE

The investigation of age as a risk factor involved the examination of data from Phases V, VII, IX and XI of the study. Referring back to the rates reported in Table 4.2, it can be seen that the prevalence of OME, as evidenced by a type B tympanogram, was greatest at the age of 5 years (10.5 per cent), decreasing to 6.5 per cent at 7 years, 3.0 per cent at 9 years and 2.4 per cent at 11 years. These findings confirm the generally held view that the risk of OME declines at around 6 or 7 years of age.

SEX

There was a significant association between sex and OME in the Dunedin sample. Examination of the data revealed that proportionately more boys than girls had had at least one episode of OME. Of the children in Groups 1, 2 and 3, 57 per cent were boys. This male preponderance was even more marked in those children with persistent bilateral OME, the ratio of boys to girls here being almost 2:1. This finding is in support of a number of previous studies which found significant sex differences in both the prevalence and duration of OME (Poulsen and Tos 1978, Tos and Poulsen 1979, Fiellau-Nikolajsen 1983*b*, Casselbrant *et al.* 1984).

RACE

Since the great majority (95.5 per cent) of the present sample were Caucasian, with the remaining 4.5 per cent comprising Maori, Polynesian and Asian children (Silva *et al.* 1981), it was considered inappropriate to investigate this factor.

SOCIO-ECONOMIC AND CULTURAL DIFFERENCES

Elley and Irving's (1972) scale of socio-economic status (SES) was used to classify the children at birth according to their father's occupation at that time. The children of solo mothers were not included in this classification, which meant the numbers available for comparison were reduced slightly. Levels one and two, three and four, and five and six of Elley and Irving's scale were each combined for this analysis. As indicated in Table 4.8, there was no significant difference between groups, indicating that OME was not significantly associated with SES levels in the present sample. This confirms the findings of Black (1985), but is at variance with the finding by Tos *et al.* (1978) of a decreased prevalence of OME among children from low-SES backgrounds. There is a need for further research on this factor.

BREAST-FEEDING

The groups differed significantly with regard to the duration of breast-feeding. Examination of the data revealed that breast-feeding for a minimum of three months appeared to protect against OME. However, this conclusion is at variance with the findings of previous studies (Kraemer *et al.* 1984, Visscher *et al.* 1984, Black 1985).

FAMILY HISTORY

This factor was not investigated in the present study.

RELATED DISORDERS

A history of ear infection, a history of sore ears, and a history of pus discharge (at Phase V only) were all associated with OME. Sore ears and purulent discharge signify acute OM, a history of which has been found to increase the risk of OME (Kaneko *et al.* 1984, Kraemer *et al.* 1984, Mills *et al.* 1986).

A history of nasal obstruction and a clinical diagnosis of nasal obstruction were both shown to be related to OME. However, there was no association between increased turbinate size and OME. The findings on nasal obstruction are consistent with previous research (Kraemer *et al.* 1984).

A history of tonsillitis was significantly associated with OME. This result is inconsistent with earlier findings reported by Tos *et al.* (1979*a*) and Van Cauwenberge (1986). No association was found between OME and either tonsil size on examination or evidence of cervical adenitis.

From the evidence reviewed earlier it is not certain what role, if any, is played by allergy in the occurrence of OME. No association was found in the present study between OME and a history of wheezing, hay fever, eczema, bronchitis or asthma. On the basis of the respiratory function tests carried out at Phase IX, no relationship was found between OME and evidence of hyper-reactive airways.

OTHER HOST FACTORS

Whereas Van Cauwenberge and Kluyskens (1984) found that low birthweight,

TABLE 4.9
Prevalence of OME (as evidenced by a type B tympanogram) in right and left ears

Phase	*Prevalence*		*Test statistic*	
	Right ear	*Left ear*		
V	93	88	$\chi^2(1df) = 0.054$	*ns*
VII	62	46	$\chi^2(1df) = 2.039$	*ns*
IX	23	24	$\chi^2(1df) = 0.003$	*ns*
XI	18	20	$\chi^2(1df) = 0.021$	*ns*

ns = not significant.

short birth length and small head circumference were significant risk factors, the data reported in Table 4.8 do not support those findings. No significant differences were obtained between groups for any of these factors or for gestational age. This is consistent with the findings of Black (1985).

Previous studies have shown that there is no difference between right and left ears in the prevalence of OME (Poulsen and Tos 1978, Tos *et al.* 1978). The prevalence rates for OME, as evidenced by a type B tympanogram, for right and left ears at Phases V, VII, IX and XI of the present study are given in Table 4.9. The results of Chi-square tests conducted at each phase indicated that there were no significant differences between the prevalence rates for OME for right and left ears.

Environmental factors

SEASON

Prevalence rates for OME, as evidenced by a type B tympanogram, by month and season are displayed in Table 4.10. For this sample, type B tympanograms were more prevalent during the winter and spring months. This finding is consistent with previously reported seasonal variations (Tos and Poulsen 1979; Fiellau-Nikolajsen 1979, 1983*b*; Lous and Fiellau-Nikolajsen 1981; Van Cauwenberge and Kluyskens 1984; Casselbrant *et al.* 1984; Rach *et al.* 1986; Holmquist *et al.* 1987).

SMOKING

The smoking habits of both parents were obtained at Phase IX. Each parent was classified as a 'non-smoker', 'ex-smoker' or 'smoker'. For smokers, the number of cigarettes smoked per day was obtained. It is apparent from the Chi-square result reported in Table 4.11, that the smoking habits of parents were not significantly associated with OME. While this result is consistent with findings reported by Van Cauwenberge and Kluyskens (1984) and Black (1985), it is at variance with the finding of Kraemer *et al.* (1984) that the risk of chronic middle-ear effusions is increased by the presence of more than one adult smoker in a household. While the evidence tends to support the conclusion that parental smoking is not a risk factor for OME, it is not unequivocal.

EXPERIENCE OF GROUP DAY-CARE AND PRESCHOOL FACILITIES

For the investigation of this factor, the children were classified as to whether or not

TABLE 4.10
Prevalence of OME (as evidenced by a type B tympanogram) at each phase by month and season

Season / *Month*	*Phase* V %	*VII* %	*IX* %	*XI* %
Autumn				
March	6.3	5.3	1.2	2.0
April	8.2	6.9	2.9	1.6
May	5.4	4.6	1.8	1.1
	(6.9)*	(5.6)*	(2.0)*	(1.7)*
Winter				
June	9.7	4.8	5.1	0.0
July	18.2	10.9	2.5	1.4
August	8.4	7.5	4.0	4.8
	(12.3)*	(7.7)*	(3.8)*	(2.0)*
Spring				
September	10.5	5.4	5.5	3.0
October	14.4	5.3	4.6	4.9
November	10.7	9.2	3.0	3.2
	(11.9)*	(6.7)*	(4.2)*	(3.7)*
Summer				
December	15.1	8.3	3.2	3.1
January†	0.0	15.0	0.0	0.0
February	3.5	2.0	0.0	1.8
	(8.4)*	(4.9)*	(1.2)*	(2.0)*

*Figures in parentheses are seasonal averages.
†Testing was not conducted during most of January due to summer holidays.

TABLE 4.11
Results from the investigation of environmental factors

Risk factor	*Test statistic*	
Parental smoking		
Mother	$\chi^2(35df) = 49.99$	*ns*
Father	$\chi^2(35df) = 21.14$	*ns*
Attendance at group day-care and preschool facilities	$\chi^2(5df) = 4.63$	*ns*
Family adversity	$\chi^2(5df) = 11.24$	*

*$p<0.05$; *ns* = not significant.

they had attended group day-care or preschool facilities before the age of 5 years. As reported in Table 4.11, there was no significant difference between groups on this factor. While confirming one previous finding (Kraemer *et al.* 1984), this result is at variance with those of Tos and Poulsen (1979), Fiellau-Nikolajsen (1983*b*) and Black (1985), who found that group day-care increased the risk of OME.

OTHER ENVIRONMENTAL FACTORS

McGee *et al.* (1984) described a measure of adversity in the child's home environment, based on the following factors: (1) low socio-economic status; (2) large family size; (3) parental separation; (4) low maternal mental ability; (5) poor maternal mental health; and (6) poor family relationships. A score of 1 is allotted on this 'family adversity index' for any of the above items which is present in that environment. The range of possible scores is 0 to 6. In the present sample, 240 families (22.9 per cent) had a score of 2 or more on this index and could therefore be considered high on adversity. 76 families (7.9 per cent) had a score of 3 or more. As indicated in Table 4.11, there was a significant association between OME and family adversity as measured by this index.

Examination of the data revealed that 28.7 per cent of the persistent bilateral OME children (Group 1 in Table 4.7) and 34.6 per cent of the persistent unilateral OME children (Group 2) came from high-adversity families, compared with 22.9 per cent of the Group 6 children (no scarred tympanic membranes, bilateral A tympanogram, OME never proven). When the persistent bilateral and persistent unilateral OME groups were combined, it was revealed that 32.3 per cent of these children came from high adversity families compared with 21.5 per cent of the remainder of the sample (χ^2, 1df=6.52, $p<0.05$).

This result suggests that where there were two or more sources of adversity in a child's home, there was an increased risk of OME occurring and persisting throughout the mid-childhood years. The presence of any one source of adversity alone, however, was insufficient to place a child at risk.

Summary

Of the host and environmental factors investigated, a number were found to be associated with OME. The risk of OME was found to be highest at the age of 5 years, after which it gradually declined. Proportionately more boys than girls were found to have had at least one episode of OME and almost twice as many boys as girls had persistent bilateral OME. Breast-feeding for a minimum of three months appeared to protect against OME. A history of ear infection, sore ears, pus discharge, nasal obstruction and tonsillitis were all found to be associated with OME, as was a clinical diagnosis of nasal obstruction. The prevalence of OME was found to be higher during the winter and spring months than in summer or autumn. Finally, the presence of two or more sources of adversity in a child's home environment was found to increase the risk of OME. In general, these findings were consistent with those of previous studies.

All other factors investigated were found not to significantly increase the risk of OME. The evidence on several of these—respiratory allergy, perinatal characteristics, parental smoking and exposure in group day-care—remains equivocal. The finding that OME is no more prevalent in the right ear than the left ear is consistent with previously reported results. The finding on socio-economic status suggests that contrary to popular belief, this may not be a significant risk factor for OME. However, the result obtained using the family adversity index suggests that it may be more appropriate in future investigations to examine the cumulative effects of a variety of possible risk factors before rejecting the influence of any single factor such as SES.

5
AUDIOLOGICAL CHARACTERISTICS

Hearing threshold levels for the complete sample

From the pure-tone audiometry conducted at Phases V, VII, IX and XI of the study, hearing threshold levels (HTLs) were obtained for the complete sample at 500, 1000, 2000 and 4000Hz. Table 5.1 contains the mean HTLs and standard deviations for each of these frequencies at each phase, and for right and left ears separately. A mean HTL across the three frequencies of 500, 1000 and 2000Hz was calculated for each ear at each phase (*cf.* Bess 1983, Fria *et al.* 1985—see Chapter 1, p. 22): the means of these 'three-frequency averages' are presented at the foot of Table 5.1. All are for the complete sample, including those children with conductive or sensorineural hearing loss, and are thus inflated, especially at Phases V and VII, the ages when middle-ear disorders were most prevalent.

It will be noted that there are variations between the means for right and left ears. Since this was not an issue of central interest to the present study, no statistical analysis of these differences is reported. It may be that this difference is an artifact of the testing procedure, given that right ears were always tested first.

The mean HTLs at 1000, 2000 and 4000Hz at Phase VII were poorer than those at Phase V. Mean HTLs at all frequencies remained relatively stable from Phase VII on, as illustrated in Figure 5.1. The poorer HTLs at 7 years of age contradict Brooks' (1979) suggestion that younger children have poorer thresholds than older children. The finding that the mean HTLs at age 5 were all better than those at the later ages tends to support the view of Northern and Downs (1978) that an attenuated impairment scale may be more appropriate for children during the first years of life.

A small number of children at each phase had HTLs poorer than 40dB. Of these, only one had a consistent binaural hearing loss poorer than 40dB at all four phases of the study. This child, whose hearing was severely impaired, was excluded from the sample for the further analysis of audiological data. All other cases of thresholds exceeding 40dB HTL were found to be either inconsistent across phases or to be unilateral at any particular phase, and all these children were retained in the sample for subsequent analyses.

Middle-ear dysfunction

The central purpose of this chapter is to describe the degree of hearing impairment associated with OME and related middle-ear disorders. For this purpose, ears were assigned to groups according to their tympanogram type. The seven tympanogram types were defined in Table 3.48 (p. 77). The 'other' category, for ears which could not be classified, has been excluded here.

The mean HTLs for each of these groups at each phase are presented in Tables 5.2 to 5.5 and are displayed graphically in Figures 5.2 to 5.5. While the tables contain data for both ears, the figures display those for the left ear only. Since, in general, the means for the two ears did not differ substantially, it was considered

TABLE 5.1
Mean hearing threshold levels (dB HTL) by frequency and phase

Frequency		*Phase V*		*Phase VII*		*Phase IX*		*Phase XI*	
		Right ear (N=895)	*Left ear (N=891)*	*Right ear (N=869)*	*Left ear (N=869)*	*Right ear (N=813)*	*Left ear (N=813)*	*Right ear (N=800)*	*Left ear (N=800)*
500Hz	*Mean*	14.39	12.93	15.79	16.48	13.99	14.75	13.57	12.88
	SD	7.97	7.17	6.83	7.07	6.64	6.53	8.37	7.42
1000Hz	*Mean*	8.71	6.54	12.14	10.52	10.56	8.97	10.30	7.46
	SD	9.51	9.37	7.76	7.42	7.53	7.31	8.87	7.96
2000Hz	*Mean*	0.37	0.78	6.87	6.55	6.47	5.68	5.40	4.90
	SD	9.81	10.21	7.72	7.42	6.96	7.06	8.20	7.64
4000Hz	*Mean*	0.97	2.28	7.38	8.27	5.60	5.18	4.84	4.24
	SD	12.44	11.85	8.25	8.33	7.92	7.46	9.04	7.30
Average over 500, 1000 and 2000Hz	*Mean*	7.93	6.83	11.47	11.10	10.26	9.77	9.76	8.41
	SD	7.99	7.80	6.41	6.63	6.09	6.16	7.63	6.76

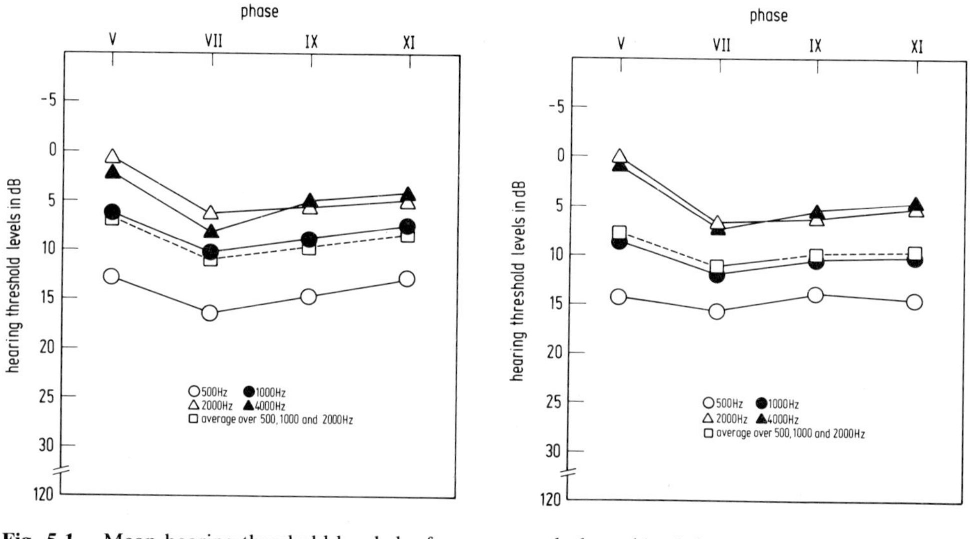

Fig. 5.1. Mean hearing threshold levels by frequency and phase (A—left ear; B—right ear).

unnecessary to display the results for both ears. The left ear was chosen because it was always tested second and due to possible learning effects, could be expected to yield less extreme values than the first tested ear.

The first point of interest is that with few exceptions the mean HTLs fall within the limits of normal hearing as defined by Green (1978), that is, –10 to 26dB HTL. As would be expected, the mean HTLs for ears in the B tympanogram group were generally poorer than those for the other groups. In four instances, the means for this group exceeded the 26dB HTL upper limit for normal hearing. When Northern and Down's (1978) scale is applied, however, almost all of the means for the B

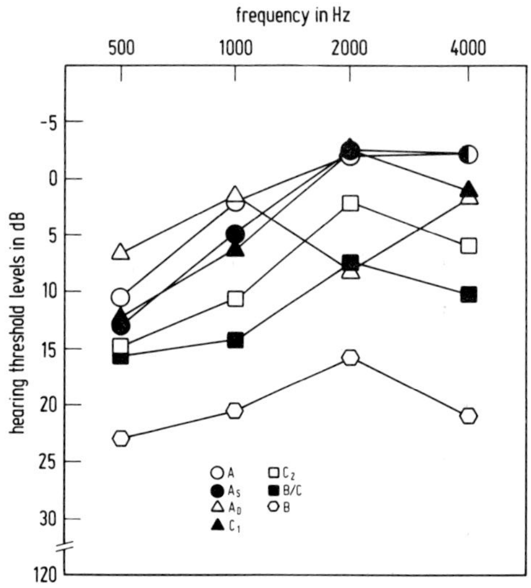

Fig. 5.2. Phase V mean hearing threshold levels by tympanogram type and frequency (left ear).

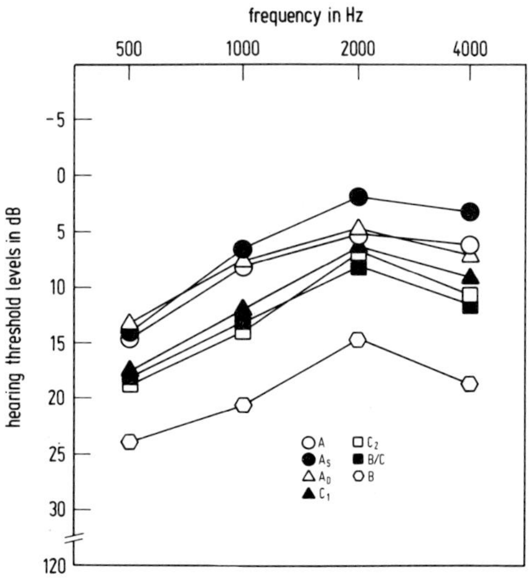

Fig. 5.3. Phase VII mean hearing threshold levels by tympanogram type and frequency (left ear).

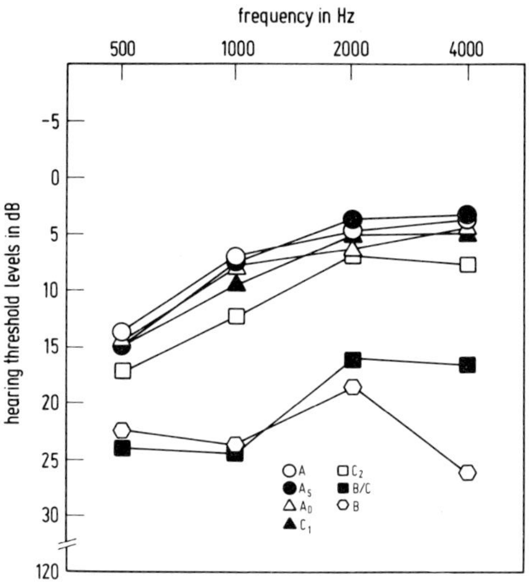

Fig. 5.4. Phase IX mean hearing threshold levels by tympanogram type and frequency (left ear).

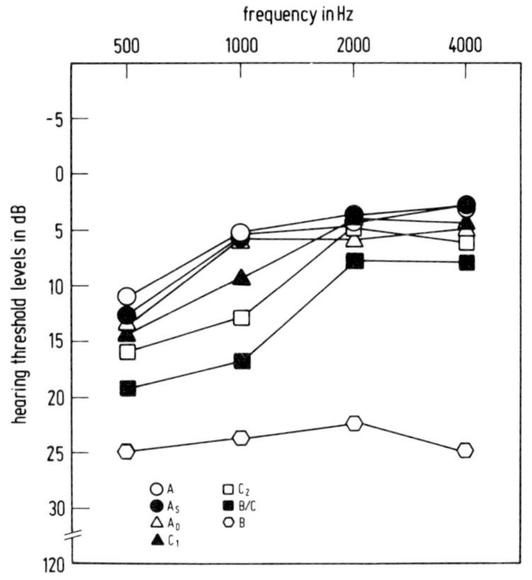

Fig. 5.5. Phase XI mean hearing threshold levels by tympanogram type and frequency (left ear).

tympanogram group fall within the 15 to 30dB HTL limits of mild hearing loss. The means also fall within the definition of hearing loss for children accepted by the New Zealand Board of Health Committee on Hearing (1984). Certainly, most fall within the range for OME identified in the literature reviewed in Chapter 1.

TABLE 5.2
Phase V mean hearing threshold levels (dB HTL) by tympanogram type and frequency

Tympanogram type	*Frequency*							
	500Hz		*1000Hz*		*2000Hz*		*4000Hz*	
	Right ear	*Left ear*	*Right ear*	*Left ear*	*Right ear*	*Left ear*	*Right ear*	*Left ear*
A	11.83	10.52	4.65	2.35	−1.82	−1.72	−3.53	−2.16
A_S	10.65	13.12	6.30	5.00	−3.04	−2.29	−3.26	−2.08
A_D	—	6.67	—	1.67	—	8.33	—	1.67
C_1	13.73	12.40	8.05	6.40	−2.07	−2.00	−0.91	1.33
C_2	15.68	14.89	11.55	10.76	0.90	2.12	4.10	6.21
B/C	18.67	15.71	18.67	14.28	5.67	7.50	6.67	10.36
B	25.64	22.74	23.20	20.55	14.62	15.75	20.32	21.10

TABLE 5.3
Phase VII mean hearing threshold levels (dB HTL) by tympanogram type and frequency

Tympanogram type	*Frequency*							
	500Hz		*1000Hz*		*2000Hz*		*4000Hz*	
	Right ear	*Left ear*	*Right ear*	*Left ear*	*Right ear*	*Left ear*	*Right ear*	*Left ear*
A	13.93	14.87	9.51	8.28	5.85	5.46	5.29	6.38
A_S	12.67	14.17	8.00	6.67	3.67	2.08	4.67	3.33
A_D	10.83	13.46	5.00	7.69	5.83	5.00	7.50	7.31
C_1	15.75	17.63	12.40	12.17	6.16	6.45	7.24	9.27
C_2	18.10	18.81	14.87	14.18	6.81	6.96	9.16	10.78
B/C	18.75	18.33	13.75	13.33	6.25	8.33	11.25	11.67
B	22.76	24.07	21.12	20.58	14.05	14.65	16.40	18.69

TABLE 5.4
Phase IX mean hearing threshold levels (dB HTL) by tympanogram type and frequency

Tympanogram type	Frequency							
	500Hz		1000Hz		2000Hz		4000Hz	
	Right ear	Left ear	Right ear	Left ear	Right ear	Left ear	Right ear	Left ear
A	12.58	13.76	8.67	7.36	5.83	5.00	4.34	3.83
A_S	14.44	15.00	10.56	7.65	4.17	3.82	3.89	3.53
A_D	12.33	14.55	9.67	7.95	6.67	6.59	4.67	4.77
C_1	15.04	14.89	11.81	9.68	6.13	5.18	5.42	5.25
C_2	16.76	17.24	14.53	12.56	6.88	7.04	8.12	7.83
B/C	19.17	24.09	19.17	24.54	10.83	16.36	5.83	16.82
B	25.94	22.50	25.94	23.75	20.62	18.75	22.81	26.25

TABLE 5.5
Phase XI mean hearing threshold levels (dB HTL) by tympanogram type and frequency

Tympanogram type	Frequency							
	500Hz		1000Hz		2000Hz		4000Hz	
	Right ear	Left ear	Right ear	Left ear	Right ear	Left ear	Right ear	Left ear
A	11.35	11.22	7.77	5.47	4.50	4.40	3.19	3.18
A_S	12.71	12.86	8.71	5.89	2.93	3.75	2.93	3.04
A_D	13.92	13.50	9.86	6.00	7.16	6.17	5.40	5.00
C_1	16.96	14.44	14.13	9.48	5.52	4.23	5.52	4.72
C_2	17.20	16.02	15.00	13.01	5.93	4.74	8.00	6.28
B/C	29.50	19.38	25.00	16.88	19.50	8.12	20.00	8.12
B	31.25	25.00	31.88	23.75	25.00	22.50	31.25	25.00

At 500Hz only, means for the C_1 and C_2 tympanogram groups were worse than the 15dB HTL lower limit for mild hearing loss. The significance of this result is questionable when it is recalled that the children were tested in a quiet but not sound-proof room.

The HTL configurations for the A tympanogram group are fairly consistent across phases, with the thresholds improving between 500 and 2000Hz, and then flattening out between 2000 and 4000Hz. Again, the apparent low-frequency loss is probably due to background noise. The configurations for the low and high compliance A type ears (types A_S and A_D) follow a similar pattern and appear to differ little in degree of loss from each other or from the A tympanogram group.

The configurations for the B tympanogram group are also relatively consistent across the four phases. Moreover, they correspond quite closely to the typical configuration for ears with OME, described by Bess (1983) as relatively flat with slight peaking at 2000Hz. The most striking feature of these configurations is the considerable gap between them and those for the remaining groups. The B/C tympanogram group was intermediate between the B and C groups.

The least consistent of the configurations are those for the C groups (C_1, C_2) and the B/C group. At Phases V and VII the C_1 configurations are similar in shape to those for the B group but closer to the type A groups in degree of loss. At Phases IX and XI they are very similar in both degree of loss and shape to the A groups. In contrast, the C_2 configurations are similar in shape to those for the B group at all phases. While they have consistently poorer thresholds than the C_1 group, they still differ from the B group by a substantial margin at all frequencies. Finally, the B/C group has a similar configuration to the C_2 group at all four phases. The degree of loss is similar for both groups at Phases V, VII and IX but there is a substantial gap between them at Phase IX, with the B/C group being closer to the B group at this phase.

In summary, it is apparent that HTLs for this sample have been adversely affected, to varying degrees, by negative middle-ear pressure and, more especially, by OME as evidenced by a type B tympanogram. In contrast, it appears that compliance outside of the normal range has had no significant effect on HTLs. To confirm these observations, a series of statistical comparisons between tympanogram groups were conducted, using methods described by Hays (1963). Both 'planned' and '*post hoc*' comparisons were performed on the data. In this form of analysis, planned comparisons are used to answer specific questions formulated before the data analysis is carried out, while *post hoc* comparisons are used to answer questions that arise after an initial analysis of the data has been conducted. The rules governing planned comparisons are more stringent than those governing *post hoc* comparisons.

Comparisons between tympanogram types

Since the primary interest here was in the effect of OME, as evidenced by a type B tympanogram, on HTLs, the first planned comparisons were made between the mean HTLs for the B tympanogram and A tympanogram groups. Comparisons were conducted for all four frequencies at each phase and for right and left ears separately. The results of these comparisons are presented in Tables 5.6 to 5.9.

TABLE 5.6
Comparisons between hearing threshold levels at Phase V

Comparisons		*Frequency*							
		500Hz		*1000Hz*		*2000Hz*		*4000Hz*	
		Right ear	*Left ear*	*Right ear*	*Left ear*	*Right ear*	*Left ear*	*Right ear*	*Left ear*
Planned									
B *vs.* A	*F*	280.25	270.21	414.68	390.17	269.00	279.41	367.03	197.32
	df	1, 852	1, 837	1, 854	1, 837	1, 853	1, 837	1, 852	1, 826
	Sig.	**	**	**	**	**	**	**	**
A_S *vs.* A_D	*F*	—	3.21	—	0.56	—	4.40	—	0.78
	df	—	1, 837	—	1, 837	—	1, 837	—	1, 826
	Sig.	—	*ns*	—	*ns*	—	*	—	*ns*
C_1 *vs.* C_2	*F*	7.00	14.96	18.45	27.43	10.97	19.12	20.24	17.47
	df	1, 852	1, 837	1, 854	1, 837	1, 853	1, 837	1, 852	1, 826
	Sig.	**	**	**	**	**	**	**	**
Remaining comparisons									
(pooled sums of squares)	*F*	2.19	1.87	9.18	17.31	3.38	3.38	5.06	11.40
	df	4, 852	4, 837	4, 854	4, 837	4, 853	4, 837	4, 852	3, 826
	Sig.	*ns*	*ns*	**	**	**	**	**	**
Post hoc									
A_S *vs.* A		—	—	*ns*	} *ns*	} *ns*	*ns*	*ns*	} *ns*
A_D *vs.* A		—	—	—	}	}	*ns*	—	}
C_1 *vs.* A		—	—	**	**	*ns*	*ns*	*ns*	*ns*
C_2 *vs.* A		—	—	**	**	*	**	**	**
B/C *vs.* A		—	—	**	**	*ns*	*	*	*ns*

*p<0.05; **p<0.01; *ns* = not significant.

TABLE 5.7
Comparisons between hearing threshold levels at Phase VII

Comparison		*Frequency*							
		500Hz		*1000Hz*		*2000Hz*		*4000Hz*	
		Right ear	*Left ear*	*Right ear*	*Left ear*	*Right ear*	*Left ear*	*Right ear*	*Left ear*
Planned									
B *vs.* A	*F*	111.19	93.04	172.90	170.71	75.14	88.32	109.58	127.45
	df	1, 826	1, 816	1, 826	1, 816	1, 816	1, 816	1, 826	1, 813
	Sig.	**	**	**	**	**	**	**	**
A_S *vs.* A_D	*F*	0.41	0.12	2.75	0.18	0.45	1.39	0.61	2.08
	df	1, 826	1, 816	1, 826	1, 816	1, 816	1, 816	1, 826	1, 813
	Sig.	*ns*	*ns*	*ns*	*ns*	**	*ns*	*ns*	*ns*
C_1 *vs.* C_2	*F*	13.13	2.25	13.04	5.70	0.79	0.40	5.40	2.78
	df	1, 826	1, 816	1, 826	1, 816	1, 826	1, 816	1, 826	1, 813
	Sig.	**	*ns*	**	*	*ns*	*ns*	*	*ns*
Remaining comparisons									
(pooled sums of squares)	*F*	9.36	11.05	15.40	24.11	1.54	1.75	3.14	7.80
	df	*3, 826*	*3, 816*	*3, 826*	*3, 816*	*3, 826*	*3, 816*	*3, 826*	*3, 813*
	Sig.	**	**	**	**	*ns*	*ns*	*	**
Post hoc									
A_S *vs.* A		} *ns*	} *ns*	} *ns*	} *ns*	—	—	} *ns*	} *ns*
A_D *vs.* A		}	}	}	}	—	—	}	}
C_1 *vs.* A		*ns*	} **	**	**	—	—	*ns*	} **
C_2 *vs.* A		**	}	**	**	—	—	**	}
B/C *vs.* A		*ns*	*ns*	*ns*	*ns*	—	—	*ns*	*ns*

*p<0.05; **p<0.01; *ns* = not significant.

TABLE 5.8
Comparisons between hearing threshold levels at Phase IX

Comparison		*Frequency*							
		500Hz		*1000Hz*		*2000Hz*		*4000Hz*	
		Right ear	*Left ear*	*Right ear*	*Left ear*	*Right ear*	*Left ear*	*Right ear*	*Left ear*
Planned									
B *vs.* A	*F*	74.87	23.42	102.87	77.80	80.88	53.40	106.37	135.11
	df	1, 778	1, 768	1, 778	1, 768	1, 778	1, 768	1, 777	1, 767
	Sig.	**	**	**	**	**	**	**	**
A_S *vs.* A_D	*F*	0.98	0.05	0.14	0.02	1.21	1.77	1.10	0.34
	df	1, 778	1, 768	1, 778	1, 768	1, 778	1, 768	1, 777	1, 767
	Sig.	*ns*	*ns*	*ns*	*ns*	*ns*	*ns*	*ns*	*ns*
C_1 *vs.* C_2	*F*	4.18	7.20	8.60	10.21	0.70	4.15	2.83	7.60
	df	1, 778	1, 768	1, 778	1, 768	1, 778	1, 768	1, 777	1, 767
	Sig.	*	**	**	**	*ns*	*	*ns*	**
Remaining comparisons									
(pooled sums of squares)	*F*	10.39	9.66	16.39	26.19	2.82	8.08	7.74	12.85
	df	4, 778	4, 768	4, 778	4, 768	4, 778	4, 768	4, 777	4, 767
	Sig.	**	**	**	**	*	**	**	**
Post hoc									
A_S *vs.* A		} *ns*	} *ns*	} *ns*	} *ns*	} *ns*	} *ns*	} *ns*	} *ns*
A_D *vs.* A		}	}	}	}	}	}	}	}
C_1 *vs.* A		*	*ns*	**	*	} *ns*	*ns*	} *	*ns*
C_2 *vs.* A		**	**	**	**	}	*ns*	}	**
B/C *vs.* A		*ns*	**	*	**	*ns*	**	*ns*	**

*p<0.05; **p<0.01; *ns* = not significant.

TABLE 5.9
Comparisons between hearing threshold levels at Phase XI

Comparison		*500Hz* Right ear	*500Hz* Left ear	*1000Hz* Right ear	*1000Hz* Left ear	*2000Hz* Right ear	*2000Hz* Left ear	*4000Hz* Right ear	*4000Hz* Left ear
		Frequency							
Planned									
B *vs.* A	*F*	57.88	51.16	84.02	89.39	66.67	86.75	104.20	122.76
	df	1, 785	1, 790	1, 785	1, 790	1, 785	1, 790	1, 785	1, 790
	Sig.	**	**	**	**	**	**	**	**
A_S *vs.* A_D	*F*	0.66	0.18	0.58	0.00	8.68	2.58	2.46	1.65
	df	1, 785	1, 790	1, 785	1, 790	1, 785	1, 790	1, 785	1, 790
	Sig.	*ns*	*ns*	*ns*	*ns*	**	*ns*	*ns*	*ns*
C_1 *vs.* C_2	*F*	0.05	2.72	0.62	13.49	0.15	0.28	4.62	2.53
	df	1, 785	1, 790	1, 785	1, 790	1, 785	1, 790	1, 785	1, 790
	Sig.	*ns*	*ns*	*ns*	**	*ns*	*ns*	*	*ns*
Remaining comparisons									
(pooled sums of squares)	*F*	33.13	14.89	39.30	25.57	13.44	1.34	20.45	3.96
	df	4, 785	4, 790	4, 785	4, 790	4, 785	4, 790	4, 785	4, 790
	Sig.	**	**	**	**	**	*ns*	**	**
Post hoc									
A_S *vs.* A		} *ns*	} *ns*	} *ns*	} *ns*	*ns*	—	} *ns*	} *ns*
A_D *vs.* A		}	}	}	}	*ns*	—	}	}
C_1 *vs.* A		} **	} **	} **	**	} *ns*	—	*ns*	} *
C_2 *vs.* A		}	}	}	**	}	—	**	}
B/C *vs.* A		*ns*	*ns*	**	**	**	—	**	*ns*

*p<0.05; **p<0.01; *ns* = not significant.

Without exception, the mean HTLs for the B group differed significantly ($p<.01$) from those for the A group.

Before making any further comparisons with the A group, the mean HTLs for the low and high compliance groups (A_S *vs.* A_D) were compared, as were those for the two negative middle-ear pressure groups (C_1 *vs.* C_2). The results of these comparisons also appear in Tables 5.6 to 5.9. With only two exceptions, the mean HTLs for the low and high compliance groups did not differ significantly. The results for the negative MEP groups, however, were not so consistent. Only at Phase V did these groups differ significantly ($p<0.01$) at all frequencies and in both ears. In those instances where the above groups did not differ significantly in this analysis, they were combined for subsequent analyses. Otherwise, they were compared with the A tympanogram group separately. One other step was taken before making these comparisons. The data were examined for evidence of further significant differences between groups by pooling the sums of squares for all remaining comparisons for each ear, at each frequency and phase. F ratios were calculated and where these were significant at $p<0.05$, *post hoc* comparisons were conducted between groups.

The mean HTLs for each of the remaining groups, at each phase and frequency, were compared with the mean HTLs for their respective tympanometrically normal counterparts. Where the foregoing planned comparisons indicated that it was appropriate to do so, groups were combined for this analysis. Again, the results of these *post hoc* comparisons are given in Tables 5.6 to 5.9.

The first point to note from these comparisons is that at no frequency for any phase did the low and high compliance groups (A_S and A_D) differ significantly from the A tympanogram group. This confirmed the impression gained from the configurations displayed in Figures 5.3 to 5.6.

As suggested earlier, no consistent overall picture of the HTLs for the C tympanogram groups has emerged from the data. Looking at the groups individually, however, some consistencies were found in the results of the *post hoc* comparisons. Firstly, for ears with MEP between –100 and –200mmH_2O (C_1), the mean HTLs were significantly poorer than the A tympanogram group at 1000Hz. The two groups did not differ at 2000Hz. These findings were consistent across all four phases. Secondly, for ears with MEP more negative than –200mmH_2O (C_2), the mean HTLs were significantly poorer than those for the A tympanogram group at 500, 1000 and 4000Hz, but not at 2000Hz, at Phases VII, IX and XI. This was not the pattern at Phase V, however, where there were significant differences at 1000, 2000 and 4000Hz, but not at 500Hz.

Finally, for the ears in the B/C tympanogram group, the mean HTLs were generally poorer than for the type A group, at Phases V, IX and XI. At Phase VII, however, the two groups did not differ significantly at any frequency.

In summary, the above results indicate that the mean HTLs for ears with evidence of OME (type B tympanograms) were significantly poorer than for tympanometrically normal ears, at all frequencies tested. The means fell largely within the range of 15 to 30dB HTL reported in previous studies. The HTL configurations over 500, 1000, 2000 and 4000Hz also followed the pattern of previous studies, being relatively flat with a slight peak at 2000Hz. Further, there

TABLE 5.10
Mean three-frequency average hearing threshold levels (dB HTL) by tympanogram type and phase

Tympanogram type	*Phase V*		*Phase VII*		*Phase IX*		*Phase XI*	
	Right ear	*Left ear*	*Right ear*	*Left ear*	*Right ear*	*Left ear*	*Right ear*	*Left ear*
A	4.87	3.72	9.55	9.45	8.93	8.65	7.88	7.03
A_S	4.63	5.28	9.00	9.58	9.61	8.65	8.12	7.50
A_D	—	5.56	6.83	8.77	9.53	9.68	10.32	8.56
C_1	6.56	5.60	11.09	11.74	11.02	9.85	12.20	9.38
C_2	9.38	9.26	13.42	13.37	12.67	12.33	12.71	11.26
B/C	14.33	12.50	13.00	13.33	16.17	21.27	24.67	14.79
B	21.15	19.68	19.66	20.84	23.38	24.00	29.38	23.75

TABLE 5.11
Mean three-frequency average hearing threshold levels (dB HTL) by tympanogram type and phase for both ears combined

Tympanogram type	*Phase V*	*Phase VII*	*Phase IX*	*Phase XI*
A	4.30	9.50	8.79	7.46
A_S	5.00	9.29	9.13	7.81
A_D	5.56	7.80	9.60	9.44
C_1	6.08	11.42	10.44	10.79
C_2	9.32	13.40	12.50	11.98
B/C	13.42	13.16	18.72	19.73
B	20.42	20.25	23.69	26.56

was no significant difference between the mean HTLs for ears with compliance either below or above the normal range of 0.3 to 1.5cm^3 and those for tympanometrically normal ears, at any of the frequencies tested at each age. No consistent pattern of mean HTLs emerged for ears with negative middle-ear pressure. It is pertinent to note that for the C_1 and C_2 groups, the mean HTLs were always better than 20dB and generally better than 15dB, particularly in the higher frequencies. The means for the B/C group exceeded 20dB HTL in the two lower frequencies at Phases IX and XI.

Three-frequency average
Green (1978) has suggested that the average HTL across the three frequencies of 500, 1000 and 2000Hz provides a satisfactory means of 'predicting the loss of sensitivity for speech'. Fria *et al.* (1985) have warned that this average 'can overestimate the true impairment for speech material in the context of OME'. It is nevertheless useful when considering the developmental consequences of OME. The HTLs used by Green for his scale of hearing impairment are based on this average.

Three-frequency average HTLs were calculated for the present sample at Phases V, VII, IX and XI. Table 5.10 presents the mean three-frequency average HTLs for both ears for each of the seven tympanogram groups at each phase.

In order to simplify the examination of these three-frequency average HTLs,

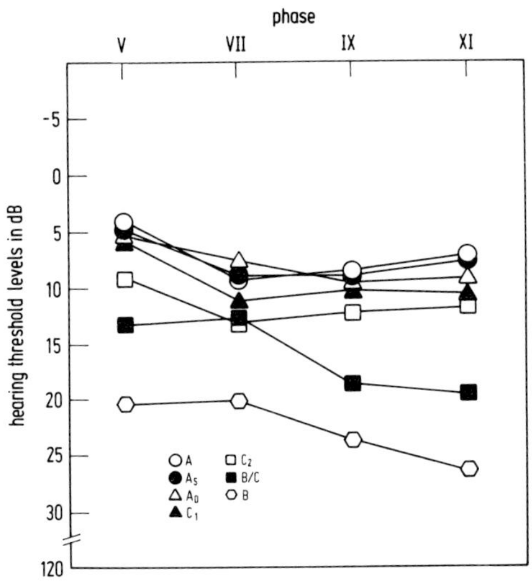

Fig. 5.6. Mean three-frequency average hearing threshold levels by tympanogram type and phase.

the data for both ears have been combined and the mean levels for each tympanogram type at each phase have been calculated. These are presented in Table 5.11 and displayed graphically in Figure 5.6.

All but one of the means shown in Table 5.11 fall within the limits of normal hearing as defined by Green. The one exception, the mean three-frequency average for the B tympanogram group at Phase XI, was slightly poorer than the 26dB HTL upper limit for normal hearing on Green's scale and fell just short of the mean of 27.6dB HTL for ears with OME described by Bess (1983). On Northern and Down's (1978) scale, the mean average HTLs for the B tympanogram group were poorer than 15dB, the lower limit for mild hearing loss, at all four phases. The mean average HTLs for the B/C tympanogram group were also poorer than 15dB, at Phases IX and XI. With the exception of Phase V, the mean average HTLs for ears with middle-ear pressure more negative than –100mmH_2O were poorer than the 10dB level predicted by Bess.

The mean three-frequency average HTLs for the A, A_S, A_D, C_1, and C_2 tympanogram groups were poorer at Phase VII than at Phase V by approximately 5dB, remaining relatively stable thereafter. This pattern is clearly illustrated in Figure 5.6, with the hearing levels for each of the above groups declining between Phases V and VII and then flattening out. It will be recalled that this pattern was observed in the mean HTLs by frequency for the complete sample (Table 5.1). In contrast, the mean average hearing levels for the B/C and B tympanogram groups were relatively stable between Phases V and VII, and then declined steadily through Phases IX and XI. This may reflect a population with more severe disease which has persisted into the older age-group.

There was little difference in mean average HTLs between the three type A groups (A, A_S, A_D), over all four phases. Moreover, the C_1 group appeared to differ little from the type A groups at any phase and the C_2 group was only marginally poorer at each phase. The substantially poorer mean average HTLs for the B/C and B tympanogram groups are clearly illustrated in Figure 5.6.

COMPARISONS BETWEEN TYMPANOGRAM TYPES

Confirmation of the above observations regarding differences between tympanogram types was made using the methods of statistical comparison described by Hays (1963) and explained earlier in this chapter. The results of this analysis are reported in Table 5.12.

As might have been expected, given the findings by frequency, the mean average HTLs for the type B group were significantly poorer than those for the type A group at all four phases. The low and high compliance groups (A_S and A_D) were not significantly different from each other and did not differ significantly from the type A group. With the exception of only one comparison, the group with middle-ear pressure between –100 and –200mmH_2O (C_1) differed significantly from the group with middle-ear pressure more negative than –200mmH_2O (C_2), thereby justifying the original separation of these two groups. The pattern of differences between the C_1 and A type ears was not consistent across phases, with those for both ears being non-significant at Phase V and significant at Phase XI. At Phases VII and IX, the differences were significant in only one ear. In contrast, the C_2 group had significantly ($p<0.01$) poorer mean average HTLs in both ears at all four phases. Finally, the mean average HTLs for the B/C group were significantly poorer than those for the type A group at Phases V and XI, did not differ significantly at Phase VII, and were inconsistent at Phase IX.

In summary, the above findings confirmed that ears with type B tympanograms, indicating OME, had significantly poorer mean three-frequency average HTLs than normal ears. The mean HTLs for ears in this group rose from 20.4dB at 5 years of age to 26.6dB at 11. For ears with abnormally low or abnormally high compliance, the mean average HTLs did not differ significantly from the A type ears at any age. The mean average HTLs for these groups never exceeded 10dB. A similar configuration was obtained for ears with middle-ear pressure more negative than -100mmH_2O, but at slightly lower levels. While the first of these groups (C_1) did not differ significantly from the type A group in any consistent manner, the second group (C_2) was consistently poorer at all four phases and exceeded 10db HTL at 7, 9 and 11 years. In contrast, the B/C group followed the pattern of the type B group, increasing from 13dB HTL at 5 and 7 years to almost 20dB HTL at 11 years.

Hearing in better ear

To obtain a better understanding of how the hearing of an individual child might be affected by OME or other middle-ear disorder, it was decided to examine the hearing threshold levels for the better ear of each member of the sample. It was believed that by using this approach a more valid indication of the disruption to communication associated with each of the middle-ear disorders, or any combination of these, might be obtained. For this purpose, children were assigned to groups according to the status of their two ears.

TABLE 5.12
Comparisons between group means for three-frequency average hearing threshold levels

Comparison		*Phase V* Right ear	*Phase V* Left ear	*Phase VII* Right ear	*Phase VII* Left ear	*Phase IX* Right ear	*Phase IX* Left ear	*Phase XI* Right ear	*Phase XI* Left ear
Planned									
B *vs.* A	*F*	475.11	469.62	197.32	188.15	109.63	94.93	89.01	102.91
	df	1, 852	1, 837	1, 826	1, 816	1, 781	1, 777	1, 785	1, 790
	Sig.	**	**	**	**	**	**	**	**
A_S *vs.* A_D	*F*	—	0.01	0.78	0.15	0.00	0.35	2.89	0.69
	df	—	1, 837	1, 826	1, 816	1, 781	1, 777	1, 785	1, 790
	Sig.	—	*ns*	*ns*	*ns*	*ns*	*ns*	*ns*	*ns*
C_1 *vs.* C_2	*F*	17.82	30.40	17.47	5.67	4.81	10.53	0.29	5.27
	df	1, 852	1, 837	1, 826	1, 816	1, 781	1, 777	1, 785	1, 790
	Sig.	**	**	**	*	*	**	*ns*	**
Remaining comparisons (pooled sums of squares)	*F*	3.85	4.32	11.40	9.10	11.23	17.04	33.12	12.47
	df	4, 852	4, 837	3, 826	3, 816	4, 781	4, 777	4, 785	4, 790
	Sig.	**	**	**	**	**	**	**	**
Post hoc									
A_S *vs.* A		*ns*	} *ns*	} *ns*	} *ns*	} *ns*	} *ns*	} *ns*	} *ns*
A_D *vs.* A		—							
C_1 *vs.* A		*ns*	*ns*	*ns*	**	**	*ns*	} **	*
C_2 *vs.* A		**	**	**	**	**	**		**
B/C *vs.* A		**	**	*ns*	*ns*	*ns*	**	**	*

*p<0.05; **p<0.01; *ns* = not significant.

TABLE 5.13
Number of children assigned to each group at each phase for analysis of audiological data for the better ear

Group	*Phase V*	*Phase VII*	*Phase IX*	*Phase XI*
Bilateral A	347	356	430	499
Bilateral B	49	13	9	10
Unilateral B	78	43	20	17
Bilateral Tubes	20	70	19	—
Unilateral Tube	6	18	8	—
Bilateral C	232	178	140	126
Unilateral C	149	177	147	138
	881	855	773	790
Missing cases	110	99	182	135
Total sample	991	954	955	925

Since it was apparent, from the comparisons reported above, that the mean HTLs by frequency of the low and high compliance types (A_S and A_D) did not differ significantly from those of the tympanometrically normal ears (type A), these three types were combined into a single type A category. To make allowance at each phase for those ears in which tympanostomy tubes had been inserted during the previous two years, a 'tubes' category was included. Because of the lack of consistency in the findings for C_1 and C_2 type ears, these groups were combined into a single type C category. Since, as reported, the B/C group was found to be intermediate between the B and C groups, and because it was desired to keep the B type ears (being those of central interest to the study) as a separate group for the present analysis, the B/C type ears were included in the C category. This was not expected to obscure any important differences in the data.

In summary, then, four categories of ear were used in the assignment of children to groups for the present analysis. These were type A, type B, 'tubes', and type C. The seven groups used in the analysis were: Bilateral A (normal); Bilateral B; Unilateral B; Bilateral Tubes; Unilateral Tube; Bilateral C; Unilateral C. In the case of the Unilateral B, Unilateral Tube and Unilateral C groups, the contralateral ear was disregarded.

The numbers of children assigned to each group at each phase are recorded in Table 5.13. As indicated by the 'missing cases' figure for each phase, a number of children were lost to this analysis because only incomplete data were available for them. Since no otological questionnaire was administered and no otological examination conducted at Phase XI, there was no record of tympanostomy tubes at this phase. From the records of the Dunedin Hospital Otolaryngology Service, however, it was known that the number of children concerned was insignificant.

Comparisons between groups

The expectation before analysing the data was that only those children in the Bilateral B and Bilateral C groups would have significantly poorer HTLs in their better ear at each frequency than for the Bilateral A group. Further, it was expected that the mean HTLs at each frequency for all of the remaining groups would tend towards the mean HTLs for the Bilateral A group.

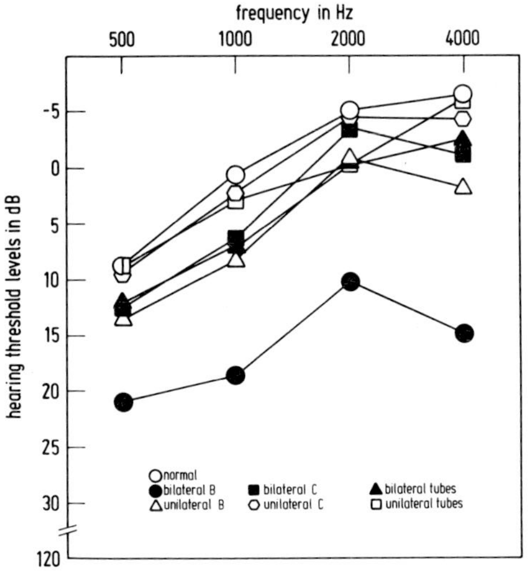

Fig. 5.7. Mean hearing threshold levels of better ear at Phase V by group and frequency.

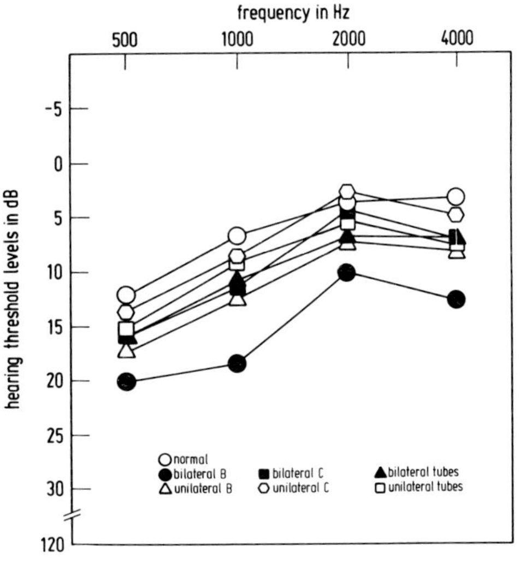

Fig. 5.8. Mean hearing threshold levels of better ear at Phase VII by group and frequency.

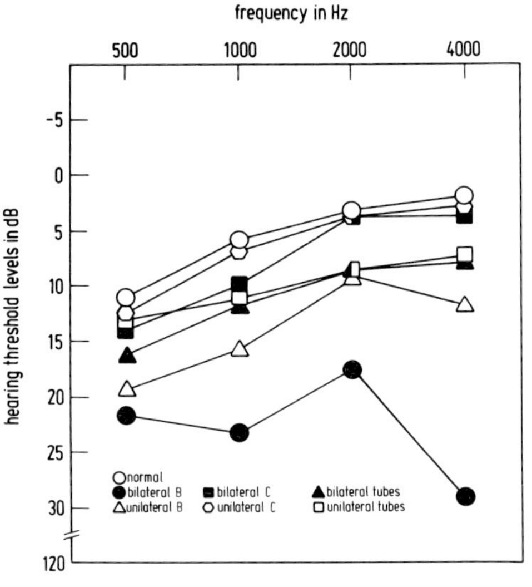

Fig. 5.9. Mean hearing threshold levels of better ear at Phase IX by group and frequency.

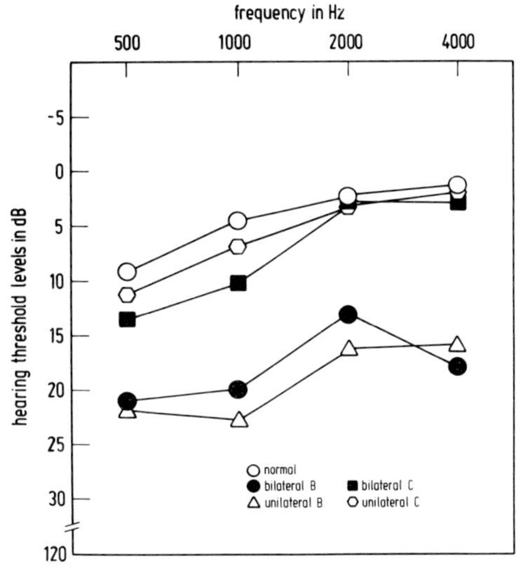

Fig. 5.10. Mean hearing threshold levels of better ear at Phase XI by group and frequency.

Tables 5.14 to 5.17 show the mean HTLs and standard deviations at 500, 1000, 2000 and 4000Hz for the 'better' ears of children in each of the above groups, for Phases V, VII, IX and XI respectively. The means are also presented graphically in Figures 5.7 to 5.10. The mean three-frequency average HTLs and standard deviations for better ears, at each phase, are set out in Table 5.18 and illustrated in Figure 5.11.

TABLE 5.14

Means and standard deviations for hearing threshold levels of better ear at Phase V by group and frequency; and group comparisons

Group	*Frequency*											
	500Hz			*1000Hz*			*2000Hz*			*4000Hz*		
	Mean		*SD*	*Mean*		*SD*	*Mean*		*SD*	*Mean*		*SD*
Bilateral A	8.93		5.13	0.73		6.02	−4.89		5.48	−6.28		5.59
Bilateral B	21.06		8.00	18.62		9.25	10.32		11.58	14.89		14.76
Unilateral B	13.57		5.18	8.31		6.52	−0.58		7.74	1.95		9.70
Bilateral Tubes	12.35		6.40	7.06		6.39	−0.29		7.17	−2.35		5.89
Unilateral Tube	9.00		6.52	3.00		4.47	0.00		5.00	−6.00		5.48
Bilateral C	12.65		6.53	6.77		8.63	−3.34		8.76	−1.00		9.63
Unilateral C	9.42		5.42	2.59		6.35	−4.24		6.86	−4.16		7.16
Planned comparisons	*F*	*df*		*F*	*df*		*F*	*df*		*F*	*df*	
Bilateral B *vs.* Bilateral A	182.62	1, 855	**	265.81	1, 855	**	179.00	1, 855	**	281.57	1, 855	**
Bilateral Tubes *vs.* Unilateral Tube	1.29	1, 855	*ns*	1.27	1, 855	*ns*	0.00	1, 855	*ns*	0.78	1, 855	*ns*
Bilateral C *vs.* Unilateral C	25.90	1, 855	**	29.02	1, 855	**	1.26	1, 855	*ns*	14.44	1, 855	**
Remaining comparisons	7.23	3, 855	**	16.04	3, 855	**	4.58	3, 855	**	10.74	3, 855	**
Post hoc *comparisons*												
Unilateral B *vs.* Bilateral A		**			**			**			**	
Bilateral Tubes *vs.* Bilateral A		} *ns*			} *ns*			} *ns*			} *ns*	
Unilateral Tube *vs.* Bilateral A		} *ns*			} *ns*			} *ns*			} *ns*	
Bilateral C *vs.* Bilateral A		**			**			} *ns*			**	
Unilateral C *vs.* Bilateral A		*ns*			*ns*			} *ns*			*ns*	

*p<0.05; **p<0.01; *ns* = not significant.

TABLE 5.15

Means and standard deviations for hearing threshold levels of better ear at Phase VII by group and frequency; and group comparisons

Group	*Frequency*											
	500Hz			*1000Hz*			*2000Hz*			*4000Hz*		
	Mean		*SD*	*Mean*		*SD*	*Mean*		*SD*	*Mean*		*SD*
Bilateral A	12.41		5.92	6.75		5.99	3.69		6.01	3.36		4.53
Bilateral B	20.00		6.12	18.46		7.47	10.00		8.42	12.69		13.32
Unilateral B	17.50		6.17	12.62		6.46	7.38		4.84	8.33		6.21
Bilateral Tubes	16.03		6.94	11.10		7.47	6.91		6.41	7.16		8.13
Unilateral Tube	15.28		4.36	9.17		4.92	5.56		5.11	7.78		7.12
Bilateral C	15.90		5.64	11.64		6.09	4.55		5.06	7.07		5.19
Unilateral C	13.75		5.54	8.69		5.21	4.12		5.29	5.08		5.74
Planned comparisons	*F*	*df*		*F*	*df*		*F*	*df*		*F*	*df*	
Bilateral B *vs.* Bilateral A	20.94	1, 842	**	47.27	1, 842	**	15.42	1, 842	**	34.22	1, 839	**
Bilateral Tubes *vs.* Unilateral Tube	0.23	1, 842	*ns*	1.47	1, 842	*ns*	0.81	1, 842	*ns*	0.17	1, 839	*ns*
Bilateral C *vs.* Unilateral C	13.44	1, 842	**	24.00	1, 842	**	0.57	1, 842	*ns*	12.45	1, 839	**
Remaining comparisons	15.88	3, 842	**	22.32	3, 842	**	9.01	3, 842	**	19.31	3, 839	**
Post hoc *comparisons*												
Unilateral B *vs.* Bilateral A		**			**			**			**	
Bilateral Tubes *vs.* Bilateral A		} *			} *			} *ns*			} **	
Unilateral Tube *vs.* Bilateral A												
Bilateral C *vs.* Bilateral A		**			**			} *ns*			**	
Unilateral C *vs.* Bilateral A		*ns*			*ns*						*ns*	

*p<0.05; **p<0.01; *ns* = not significant.

TABLE 5.16

Means and standard deviations for hearing threshold levels of better ear at Phase IX by group and frequency; and group comparisons

Group	*Frequency*											
	500Hz			*1000Hz*			*2000Hz*			*4000Hz*		
	Mean		*SD*	*Mean*		*SD*	*Mean*		*SD*	*Mean*		*SD*
Bilateral A	11.02		5.09	5.87		4.50	3.42		4.61	2.09		3.62
Bilateral B	21.67		6.06	23.33		4.08	17.50		5.24	29.17		10.68
Unilateral B	19.38		6.23	15.62		8.63	9.38		7.76	11.88		7.53
Bilateral Tubes	16.32		8.79	11.84		9.46	8.68		9.26	7.89		8.55
Unilateral Tube	13.12		6.51	11.25		7.44	8.75		8.34	7.50		8.02
Bilateral C	14.21		5.90	9.96		6.82	3.81		4.57	3.92		4.69
Unilateral C	12.59		4.78	6.92		5.14	3.81		4.59	2.99		4.50
Planned comparisons	*F*	*df*		*F*	*df*		*F*	*df*		*F*	*df*	
Bilateral B *vs.* Bilateral A	23.31	1, 740	**	62.16	1, 740	**	49.43	1, 740	**	225.26	1, 739	**
Bilateral Tubes *vs.* Unilateral Tube	1.99	1, 740	*ns*	0.07	1, 740	*ns*	0.00	1, 740	*ns*	0.04	1, 739	*ns*
Bilateral C *vs.* Unilateral C	6.55	1, 740	*	22.28	1, 740	**	0.00	1, 740	*ns*	3.23	1, 739	*ns*
Remaining comparisons	16.96	3, 740	**	20.39	3, 740	**	12.79	3, 740	**	24.59	3, 739	**
Post hoc *comparisons*												
Unilateral B *vs.* Bilateral A		**			**			*ns*			**	
Bilateral Tubes *vs.* Bilateral A		} *ns*			} **			} **			} **	
Unilateral Tube *vs.* Bilateral A		} *ns*			} **			} **			} **	
Bilateral C *vs.* Bilateral A		**			**			} *ns*			} *	
Unilateral C *vs.* Bilateral A		*ns*			*ns*			} *ns*			} *	

*p<0.05; **p<0.01; *ns* = not significant.

TABLE 5.17
Means and standard deviations for hearing threshold levels of better ear at Phase XI by group and frequency; and group comparisons

Group	*Frequency*											
	500Hz			*1000Hz*			*2000Hz*			*4000Hz*		
	Mean		*SD*	*Mean*		*SD*	*Mean*		*SD*	*Mean*		*SD*
Bilateral A	9.23		5.83	4.48		6.08	2.69		5.70	1.58		3.41
Bilateral B	21.00		9.62	20.00		12.75	13.00		9.75	18.00		10.37
Unilateral B	21.67		10.61	22.78		10.34	16.11		15.77	16.11		18.81
Bilateral Tubes	—		—	—		—	—		—	—		—
Unilateral Tube	—		—	—		—	—		—	—		—
Bilateral C	13.53		5.78	10.31		6.27	2.83		4.59	3.14		4.55
Unilateral C	11.30		6.72	6.92		6.58	3.26		5.19	2.44		4.61
Planned comparisons	*F*	*df*		*F*	*df*		*F*	*df*		*F*	*df*	
Bilateral B *vs.* Bilateral A	18.75	1, 766	**	30.21	1, 766	**	16.49	1, 766	**	71.21	1, 765	**
Bilateral Tubes *vs.* Unilateral Tube	—	—	—	—	—	—	—	—	—	—	—	—
Bilateral C *vs.* Unilateral C	8.97	1, 766	**	20.74	1, 766	**	0.09	1, 766	*ns*	1.29	1, 765	*ns*
Remaining comparisons	37.84	2, 766	**	67.12	2, 766	**	24.30	2, 766	**	50.74	2, 765	**
Post hoc *comparisons*												
Unilateral B *vs.* Bilateral A		**			**			**			**	
Bilateral Tubes *vs.* Bilateral A		—			—			—			—	
Unilateral Tube *vs.* Bilateral A		—			—			—			—	
Bilateral C *vs.* Bilateral A		**			**			} *ns*			} *	
Unilateral C *vs.* Bilateral A		*ns*			*			}			}	

*p<0.05; **p<0.01; *ns* = not significant.

TABLE 5.18
Means and standard deviations for three-frequency average hearing threshold levels of better ear by group and phase; and group comparisons

Group	Phase V Mean	Phase V SD	Phase VII Mean	Phase VII SD	Phase IX Mean	Phase IX SD	Phase XI Mean	Phase XI SD
Bilateral A	2.37	4.39	8.02	5.31	7.24	3.88	6.01	5.22
Bilateral B	17.41	8.58	16.31	6.77	21.83	4.49	18.00	10.50
Unilateral B	7.38	4.93	12.74	5.20	15.00	5.68	20.18	11.47
Bilateral Tubes	6.57	5.05	11.52	5.80	13.21	9.68	—	—
Unilateral Tube	5.00	4.08	10.56	4.58	11.62	6.70	—	—
Bilateral C	5.77	5.08	10.99	4.67	9.77	4.96	9.44	4.73
Unilateral C	3.34	5.07	9.47	5.22	8.14	4.11	7.63	5.45

	Phase V F	Phase V df		Phase VII F	Phase VII df		Phase IX F	Phase IX df		Phase XI F	Phase XI df	
Planned comparisons												
Bilateral B *vs.* Bilateral A	369.46	1, 854	**	31.63	1, 841	**	64.02	1, 742	**	25.30	1, 766	**
Bilateral Tubes *vs.* Unilateral Tube	0.37	1, 854	*ns*	0.48	1, 841	*ns*	0.72	1, 742	*ns*	—	—	—
Bilateral C *vs.* Unilateral C	19.29	1, 854	**	7.73	1, 841	**	9.70	1, 742	**	7.69	1, 766	**
Remaining comparisons	8.96	3, 854	**	17.38	3, 841	**	21.33	3, 742	**	45.54	2, 766	**
Post hoc *comparisons*												
Unilateral B *vs.* Bilateral A		**			**			**			**	
Bilateral Tubes *vs.* Bilateral A		} *ns*			} *			} **			—	
Unilateral Tube *vs.* Bilateral A		}			}			}			—	
Bilateral C *vs.* Bilateral A		**			**			**			**	
Unilateral C *vs.* Bilateral A		*ns*			*ns*			*ns*			*ns*	

*p<0.05; **p<0.01; *ns* = not significant.

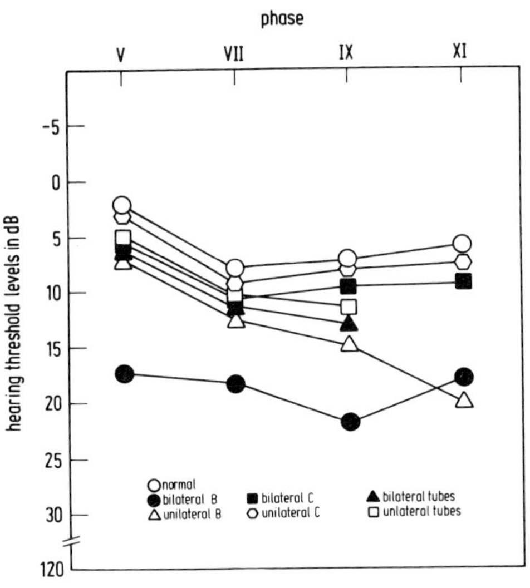

Fig. 5.11. Mean three-frequency average hearing threshold levels of better ear by group and phase.

METHOD OF ANALYSIS

The overall objective of this analysis was to determine if the mean HTLs for any of the six abnormal groups differed significantly from the mean HTLs for the Bilateral A group. Again, the method of planned and *post hoc* comparisons described by Hays (1963) and explained earlier in this chapter was used. Since it was predicted that the Bilateral B group would differ significantly from the Bilateral A group, planned comparisons between the means for these groups were conducted for each of the four frequencies at each phase and for the three-frequency average at each phase. Planned comparisons were then conducted between the Bilateral Tubes and Unilateral Tube groups and the Bilateral C and Unilateral C groups for each of the frequencies and for the three-frequency average at each phase. These analyses were conducted primarily for the purpose of deciding whether or not either of these pairs of groups should be combined for subsequent comparisons. The sums of squares for all remaining comparisons were then pooled and F ratios calculated to determine if there were any further significant differences between groups. Finally, with groups being combined as appropriate, the remaining groups were compared with the Bilateral A group, using the *post hoc* method. The results of these analyses are presented beneath the means and standard deviations in Tables 5.14 to 5.18.

BILATERAL B GROUP

The mean HTLs by frequency for the better ear of children in the Bilateral B group followed the expected pattern. The configurations for this group were of the now familiar shape, being relatively flat with slight peaking at 2000Hz. It is of interest that at Phases V, VII and XI the mean HTLs did not exceed 15dB at 2000Hz and, similarly, at Phases V and VII did not exceed 15dB at 4000Hz. This was not the case at Phase IX, which suggests that the effects of OME, as evidenced by a type B tympanogram, were greatest at this age. In general, however, the means were 3 to 4dB HTL better than those reported earlier. The planned comparisons indicate that the Bilateral B group differed significantly ($p<0.01$) from the Bilateral A group at all frequencies and at all phases. The mean three-frequency average HTLs for the Bilateral B group were all significantly poorer than normal (Table 5.18). Nevertheless, they were better than 20dB at Phases V, VII and XI, and exceeded this figure by less than 2dB at Phase IX. It is important to recall from Table 5.13 that the numbers of children with bilateral B tympanograms at ages 9 and 11 were small.

COMPARISONS AT PHASE V

At Phase V the mean HTLs by frequency in the better ear for all groups other than the Bilateral B group tended towards the mean HTLs for children in the Bilateral A, or 'normal' group. The comparisons reported in Table 5.14 indicated that, for the Unilateral B group, the mean HTLs at all frequencies were significantly poorer than those for the Bilateral A group. No mean HTL, however, exceeded 15dB at any frequency. Similarly, the comparisons for the Bilateral C group indicated that the mean HTLs were significantly poorer than the Bilateral A group at all but 2000Hz, at which frequency there was no significant difference. While this finding supported the earlier prediction, again the mean HTLs did not exceed 15dB. The Bilateral and Unilateral Tube groups did not differ significantly from each other or from the Bilateral A group at any frequency. Similarly, the Unilateral C group did not differ significantly from the Bilateral A group at any frequency. The comparisons reported in Table 5.18 for the mean three-frequency average HTLs were consistent with the above pattern. At Phase V, the mean HTLs did not exceed 10dB for any group, with the exception of the Bilateral B group. The only unexpected finding, therefore, was for the Unilateral B group. The mean HTLs for this group were poorer than expected, suggesting that a substantial number of these children may have had other than type A tympanograms in their better ear at the time of testing.

COMPARISONS AT PHASE VII

The differences between the groups were less pronounced at Phase VII (Table 5.15). While the configuration of mean HTLs by frequency for the Bilateral B group differed little from that obtained at Phase V, all other configurations were poorer overall than those for the previous phase. This, of course, reflects the overall change in HTLs between ages 5 and 7, described earlier. The mean HTLs for all but the Bilateral B group remained better than 15dB at 1000, 2000 and 4000Hz, while at 500Hz they ranged from 13.75 to 17.50dB. Apart from this change in degree of hearing loss, the overall pattern differed little from that at Phase V. One difference which did occur was that the mean HTLs for the Bilateral and Unilateral Tube groups were significantly poorer than the Bilateral A group at 500, 1000 and 4000Hz. They exceeded 15dB HTL, however, at only 500 Hz. Again, the comparisons for the mean three-frequency average HTLs, as reported in Table 5.18, were consistent with this pattern.

COMPARISONS AT PHASE IX

At Phase IX, the numbers of children assigned to the 'abnormal' groups dropped markedly, with the exception of the Bilateral and Unilateral C groups which still contained substantial numbers. As Table 5.16 indicates, the mean HTLs by frequency for the Bilateral B group were somewhat poorer than for the previous two phases, particularly in the higher frequencies. The general pattern of differences between the remaining groups and the Bilateral A group were relatively unchanged, as indicated in Figure 5.9. An interesting trend became apparent, however, when the mean three-frequency average HTLs for this phase, as presented in Table 5.18 and Figure 5.11, were examined. Whereas the mean average HTLs for the Bilateral A, Bilateral C and Unilateral C groups had improved slightly between Phase VII and Phase IX, those for the Unilateral B, Bilateral Tubes and Unilateral Tube groups were all poorer at Phase IX than at Phase VII. For none of these groups, however, did mean HTLs exceed 15dB.

COMPARISONS AT PHASE XI

The mean HTLs by frequency for the Bilateral B group at Phase XI were similar to those obtained at Phases V and VII (Table 5.17, Fig. 5.10). The mean HTLs for the two type C tympanogram groups were very similar to those obtained at Phase IX. The results for Phase XI differed, however, from those for all previous phases with respect to the Unilateral B group. At all but 4000Hz the mean HTLs for this group were poorer than those for the Bilateral B group. When the mean three-frequency average HTLs for the Unilateral B group were examined (Table 5.18, Fig. 5.11), it was apparent that the downward trend first evidenced at Phase VII had continued through Phases IX and XI.

Summary

The hearing threshold levels of the 'better' ears of the children in the sample were examined, in the belief that this would provide a more valid description of the actual hearing loss suffered by children with OME or MEP more negative than –100mmH_2O.

The mean HTLs by frequency of the better ear of the children in the Bilateral B group were 3 to 4dB better than the means for both ears reported earlier. Generally, the mean HTLs were poorer at 500 and 1000Hz, ranging from 18 to 23dB, while at 2000 and 4000Hz they were often better than 15dB. The mean three-frequency average HTLs were generally better than 20dB, ranging from 16 to 22dB.

For children in the Unilateral B group, there was a trend over the four phases for the mean HTLs by frequency of the better ear to become poorer. This was clearly seen in the mean three-frequency average HTLs, which declined steadily from 7dB at Phase V to 20dB at Phase XI.

For those children who had had tympanostomy tubes inserted either bilaterally or unilaterally in the previous two years, the mean HTLs by frequency of the better ear were similar to the Bilateral A group at Phase V. Although significantly poorer than that group at Phases VII and IX, the mean HTLs were better than 15dB at all but 500Hz.

Finally, the mean HTLs by frequency of the better ear of children in the Bilateral C group were significantly poorer than those for the Bilateral A group at 500, 1000 and 4000Hz but not at 2000Hz. The mean HTLs for the Unilateral C group generally did not differ significantly from those for the Bilateral A group.

6
DEVELOPMENTAL CONSEQUENCES

Introduction

Two different approaches were taken in the investigation of the developmental consequences of hearing loss secondary to OME in the Dunedin sample. The first involved the *cross-sectional* analysis of data collected at each phase of the study. In this approach, children at each phase who had evidence of OME were compared on a variety of developmental measures with those children at the same phase who had type A tympanograms bilaterally. Similarly, since at least one previous study (Cook and Teel 1979) had reported an association between developmental delays and negative middle-ear pressure, children in the Dunedin sample with MEP more negative than –100mmH_2O were compared with the bilateral A group.

Whereas the approach described above involved separate and independent analyses of the data collected at each phase of the study, the second approach involved a *longitudinal* analysis of the data collected over all phases of the study. In this approach, children with evidence of OME at Phase V and those with otologically normal ears at this phase were compared in terms of their performance over the five phases of the study on a variety of developmental measures. Children with MEP more negative than –100mmH_2O were not included in this analysis.

Design issues

This investigation was hampered by two main factors. To begin with, the first otological examination of the sample was made when the children were 5 years of age. This meant that there was no reliable history of the disease in any child prior to this age. And secondly, children diagnosed as having OME at the time of examination were referred for specialist otological care. It had to be accepted, therefore, that intervention at this stage could benefit the child and alleviate any long-term adverse effect that OME might have on development.

Despite the lack of a history of OME in the sample at Phase V, it was assumed that children presenting with evidence of OME at the time of examination had suffered from the disease for at least a short time prior to visiting the Study Centre.

Similarly, it was assumed that children who presented with MEP more negative than –100mmH_2O at Phase V had suffered from this condition for at least a short time prior to visiting the Unit. The time of onset, duration or frequency of occurrence of the condition, however, were not known.

Cross-sectional analysis

For the cross-sectional analysis the children were each assigned to one of the seven groups defined in Chapter 5 (p. 110): Bilateral A, Bilateral B, Unilateral B, Bilateral Tubes, Unilateral Tube, Bilateral C or Unilateral C.

Phase V results

For the investigation of the developmental consequences of OME at 5 years the

TABLE 6.1
Means and standard deviations for developmental measures at Phase III

Group (at Phase V)	*Intelligence*		*Verbal comprehension*		*Verbal expression*	
	Mean	*SD*	*Mean*	*SD*	*Mean*	*SD*
Bilateral A	23.86	9.42	35.59	8.54	36.46	8.44
Bilateral B	22.04	8.86	32.83	8.19	33.89	6.52
Unilateral B	21.77	9.57	34.60	7.67	36.10	6.58
Bilateral Tubes	21.68	10.96	30.60	10.48	34.26	9.37
Unilateral Tube	23.80	13.37	29.33	13.91	31.83	6.37
Bilateral C	23.32	9.35	34.44	8.68	36.05	8.27
Unilateral C	24.36	8.98	35.73	8.10	35.89	8.40

following measures administered at Phases III and V of the study were used. Those administered at Phase III were included because the middle-ear problems identified at Phase V could have occurred at any time between birth and 5 years.

At Phase III:

1. Intelligence—Peabody Picture Vocabulary Test;
2. Verbal comprehension—Reynell Developmental Language Scales;
3. Verbal expression—Reynell Developmental Language Scales.

At Phase V:

1. Intelligence—Stanford–Binet Intelligence Scale;
2. Verbal comprehension—Reynell Developmental Language Scales;
3. Verbal expression—Reynell Developmental Language Scales;
4. Speech articulation—Dunedin Articulation Screening Scale;
5. Behaviour problems—Rutter Child Scales A (parents) and B (teachers).

The mean scores and standard deviations for each of the seven groups on each of the above measures are presented in Tables 6.1 and 6.2.

The first step in examining these data was to determine if the Bilateral B group differed from the Bilateral Tubes group on any of the measures. The reason for making this comparison was that both the recording of a type B tympanogram and a history of tubes were taken as evidence of OME. The method of 'planned comparisons' described by Hays (1963) and explained in Chapter 5 (p. 100) was used to compare the mean scores of the two groups. The results of these comparisons are presented in the first three columns of Table 6.3. There was no significant difference between the two groups on any of the measures. It was considered appropriate, therefore, to combine these groups into one Bilateral B/Tubes group for subsequent analyses.

The next task was to see if the combined Bilateral B/Tubes group differed significantly from the Bilateral A group on any of the developmental measures. The results of these comparisons are presented in columns four to six of Table 6.3. They indicate that the Bilateral B/Tubes group had significantly lower intelligence scores at age 5 but not at age 3, had significantly lower verbal comprehension and verbal expression scores at both ages 3 and 5, and significantly higher scores on teacher-reported behaviour problems at age 5. There was no significant difference between the Bilateral B/Tubes group and the Bilateral A group on the measures of speech articulation and parent-reported behaviour problems at age 5.

TABLE 6.2
Means and standard deviations for developmental measures at Phase V

Group (at Phase V)	*Intelligence*		*Verbal comprehension*		*Verbal expression*		*Speech articulation*		*Behaviour problems** *Parents*		*Teachers*	
	Mean	*SD*	*Mean*	*SD*	*Mean*	*SD*	*Mean*	*SD*	*Mean*	*SD*	*Mean*	*SD*
Bilateral A	106.91	16.36	51.18	5.42	50.26	7.16	17.63	3.91	6.09	3.58	3.14	3.62
Bilateral B	99.83	15.40	49.23	5.28	49.40	5.78	16.34	4.86	7.57	3.01	4.62	4.38
Unilateral B	105.70	15.36	50.58	4.41	50.28	5.74	17.34	4.26	6.12	3.95	3.43	3.95
Bilateral Tubes	98.60	15.38	49.45	5.48	46.75	8.26	16.79	4.84	6.45	4.44	4.10	4.12
Unilateral Tube	103.83	26.13	50.17	2.48	50.33	7.34	16.50	4.89	7.50	4.55	4.50	3.27
Bilateral C	105.96	15.23	51.20	4.58	50.81	5.49	17.58	3.65	6.05	3.66	3.02	3.80
Unilateral C	108.29	16.88	51.60	4.25	50.48	6.36	17.28	4.14	6.59	4.09	3.41	3.56

*A higher score indicates more behaviour problems.

TABLE 6.3
Comparisons between means for developmental measures at Phases III and V

Developmental measure	*Bilateral B* vs. *Bilateral Tubes* *F*	*df*	*Sig.*	*Average of Bilateral B and Bilateral Tubes* vs. *Bilateral A* *F*	*df*	*Sig.*	*All other comparisons (pooled sum of squares)* *F*	*df*	*Sig.*
Phase III									
Intelligence	0.02	1, 826	*ns*	2.10	1, 826	*ns*	0.98	4, 826	*ns*
Verbal comprehension	0.96	1, 865	*ns*	10.09	1, 865	**	0.97	4, 865	*ns*
Verbal expression	0.03	1, 865	*ns*	4.01	1, 865	*	0.68	4, 865	*ns*
Phase V									
Intelligence	0.08	1, 869	*ns*	11.03	1, 869	**	0.99	4, 869	*ns*
Verbal comprehension	0.03	1, 872	*ns*	6.77	1, 872	**	1.21	4, 872	*ns*
Verbal expression	2.40	1, 872	*ns*	5.56	1, 872	*	0.12	4, 872	*ns*
Speech articulation	0.18	1, 865	*ns*	3.35	1, 865	*ns*	0.55	4, 865	*ns*
Behaviour problems									
Parent report	1.29	1, 870	*ns*	3.05	1, 870	*ns*	1.23	4, 870	*ns*
Teacher reports	0.27	1, 858	*ns*	4.97	1, 858	*	1.04	4, 858	*ns*

*$p<0.05$; **$p<0.01$; *ns* = not significant.

Finally, to determine if other significant differences were present in the data, the sums of squares for all remaining comparisons between groups were pooled for each of the developmental measures and F ratios calculated (Hays 1963). The purpose of this statistical procedure is to test for any significant differences between groups, out of all the possible comparisons remaining after planned comparisons have been made. In the present analysis there were seven groups of subjects, allowing for a possible 21 comparisons to be made. Since two planned comparisons had already been made, a total of 19 possible comparisons remained. Of these, the main interest was in whether the Unilateral B, Unilateral Tube or either of the negative MEP groups differed significantly from the Bilateral A group. The results of the nine F tests are contained in columns seven to nine of Table 6.3. It was evident from these results that there were no significant differences between groups for the remaining possible comparisons. If any of these F tests had been significant, then separate *post hoc* tests could have been conducted on those of the remaining 19 comparisons in which there was interest. However, as none of the F tests were significant, *post hoc* comparisons were unnecessary.

Phase VII results

The first step taken in analysing the data obtained at Phase VII was to establish whether there were any significant differences between the developmental consequences of OME occurring before the age of 5 years and the developmental consequences of OME occurring between the ages of 5 and 7 years. In other words the question asked was, are the presumed deleterious effects of OME more pronounced for those children with early onset of the disease (before 5 years of age) than for those with later onset (after 5 years)? To examine this question, children with evidence of bilateral OME at Phase VII (N=83) were separated into those first identified at Phase V and those first identified at Phase VII. As before, both the recording of bilateral B tympanograms and a history of tubes bilaterally were taken as evidence of bilateral OME. Table 6.4 presents the distribution of children with evidence of OME at Phase VII by groups and by the age at which the disease was first identified.

The developmental measures administered at Phase VII were as follows.

1. Intelligence—Wechsler Intelligence Scale for Children (WISC): Verbal Scale, Performance Scale, Full Scale.
2. Verbal comprehension—Illinois Test of Psycholinguistic Abilities (ITPA): Auditory Reception Scale.
3. Verbal expression—ITPA: Verbal Expression Scale.
4. Speech articulation—Dunedin Articulation Check.
5. Reading—Burt Word Reading Test.
6. Behaviour problems—Rutter Child Scales A (parents) and B (teachers).

Separate one-way ANOVAs were conducted for each of these measures, with age at identification as the independent variable in each case. The results of the analyses are presented in Table 6.5. Since there were no significant differences between the groups, it was clear that children for whom onset had been first recorded at the age of 5 years performed no differently to those for whom it had been recorded at the later age of 7 years.

TABLE 6.4
Age at identification for children with bilateral OME at Phase VII

Group	*Age at identification* 5 years N	7 years N	*Total*
Bilateral B	6	7	13
Bilateral Tubes	52	18	70
Total	58	25	83

TABLE 6.5
Developmental measures by age at identification at Phase VII

Developmental measure	*Age at identification* 5 years Mean	7 years Mean	*ANOVA** F	df
Intelligence				
Verbal	101.88	103.25	0.13	1, 80
Performance	104.00	104.75	0.04	1, 80
Full scale	103.21	104.25	0.08	1, 80
Verbal comprehension	27.83	26.88	0.24	1, 81
Verbal expression	26.09	29.04	1.68	1, 81
Speech articulation	14.07	13.33	0.55	1, 79
Word reading	25.88	25.92	0.00	1, 81
Behaviour problems				
Parent reports	7.77	8.84	0.87	1, 80
Teacher reports	4.81	3.60	1.05	1, 81

*All comparisons non-significant.

Having established this, the data for the seven groups and nine measures were examined using the same procedure as that described for the analysis of the Phase V data. The means and standard deviations for these data are presented in Table 6.6 and the results of the analyses in Table 6.7.

As for Phase V, the first step in this analysis involved the comparison of the Bilateral B and Bilateral Tubes groups on each of the measures. As the first three columns of Table 6.7 indicate, there were no significant differences between these groups on the measures of intelligence (verbal, performance and full scale), speech articulation, word reading, or behaviour problems (parent and teacher scales). The Bilateral B and Bilateral Tubes groups were therefore combined and compared with the Bilateral A group on these measures.

There were, however, significant differences between the two groups on the measures of verbal comprehension ($F=4.70$; $df=1, 847$; $p<0.05$) and verbal expression ($F=5.83$; $df=1, 847$; $p<0.05$). For these measures, separate *post hoc* comparisons (Scheffe 1953) were conducted between the Bilateral B and Bilateral A groups, and between the Bilateral A and Bilateral Tubes groups. The results are detailed in columns four to six of Table 6.7. Only one significant difference was obtained, the Bilateral Tubes group having a significantly lower mean score than the Bilateral A group on the measure of verbal expression ($F=13.78$; $df=1, 847$; $p<0.05$).

TABLE 6.6
Means and standard deviations for developmental measures at Phase VII

Group (at Phase VII)	*Intelligence*						*Verbal comprehension*		*Verbal expression*		*Speech articulation*		*Word reading*		*Behaviour problems**			
	Verbal		*Performance*		*Full scale*										*Parents*		*Teachers*	
	Mean	*SD*	*Mean*	*SD*	*Mean*	*SD*	*Mean*	*SD*	*Mean*	*SD*	*Mean*	*SD*	*Mean*	*SD*	*Mean*	*SD*	*Mean*	*SD*
Bilateral A	106.50	15.43	107.91	14.30	107.91	14.48	29.67	8.20	30.14	8.18	14.58	3.55	30.28	13.58	6.95	4.47	3.36	4.12
Bilateral B	109.62	12.65	106.31	11.61	109.00	11.71	32.00	4.80	32.23	8.68	14.85	3.31	29.69	9.08	7.46	4.98	3.15	3.39
Unilateral B	101.36	15.86	104.02	12.16	102.95	13.76	27.57	8.79	29.26	9.40	14.14	3.82	25.64	13.71	7.78	6.22	4.62	5.68
Bilateral Tubes	100.90	15.72	103.83	15.68	102.48	15.23	26.71	8.34	26.00	9.45	13.66	4.18	25.18	13.34	8.22	4.77	4.68	5.15
Unilateral Tube	103.50	13.51	105.61	13.23	105.61	13.56	26.61	7.39	26.94	5.92	13.44	3.54	25.78	12.57	7.50	5.62	7.39	5.34
Bilateral C	106.32	13.78	107.80	14.05	107.80	13.60	29.11	8.03	29.11	8.00	14.44	3.54	30.21	12.86	7.62	4.43	3.74	4.40
Unilateral C	106.45	13.99	107.44	14.75	107.62	14.14	28.90	7.88	30.70	9.41	14.43	3.58	29.24	12.90	6.88	4.45	4.18	4.92

*A higher score indicates more behaviour problems.

TABLE 6.7
Comparisons between means for developmental measures at Phases VII

Developmental measure	*Bilateral B* vs. *B and Bilat.*			*Average of Bilateral B and Bilateral Tubes* vs. *Bilateral A*			*All other comparisons (pooled sums of squares)*		
	F	*df*	*Sig.*	*F*	*df*	*Sig.*	*F*	*df*	*Sig.*
Intelligence									
Verbal	3.83	1, 845	*ns*	0.27	1, 845	*ns*	2.49	4, 742	*
Performance	0.33	1, 846	*ns*	1.51	1, 846	*ns*	1.40	4, 846	*ns*
Full scale	2.32	1, 845	*ns*	0.90	1, 845	*ns*	2.48	4, 845	*
Verbal comprehension	4.70	1, 847	*	(1.05	1, 847	*ns*)†	1.60	4, 847	*ns*
				(7.82	1, 847	*ns*)‡			
Verbal expression	5.83	1, 847	*	(0.75	1, 847	*ns*)†	2.90	4, 847	*
				(13.78	1, 847	*)‡			
Speech articulation	1.15	1, 843	*ns*	0.30	1, 843	*ns*	1.02	4, 843	*ns*
Word reading	1.28	1, 845	*ns*	1.78	1, 845	*ns*	2.76	4, 845	*
Behaviour problems									
Parent reports	0.03	1, 834	*ns*	1.43	1, 834	*ns*	1.47	4, 834	*ns*
Teacher reports	1.25	1, 842	*ns*	0.58	1, 842	*ns*	4.52	4, 842	**

*$p<0.05$; **$p<0.01$; *ns* = not significant.
†*Post hoc* comparison: Bilateral B *vs.* Bilateral A; ‡*Post hoc* comparison: Bilateral Tubes *vs.* Bilateral A.

As before, the final step in analysing these data involved pooling the sums of squares for all remaining comparisons for each measure. The results of these analyses are summarized in columns seven to nine of Table 6.7. Significant F tests resulted for verbal IQ, full-scale IQ, verbal expression, word reading (all at $p<0.05$), and teacher-reported behaviour problems ($p<0.01$). Separate *post hoc* comparisons revealed, however, that at a significance level of $p \leq 0.01$, an appropriately conservative criterion for this anaylsis, none of the remaining differences between groups were significant.

Phase IX results

By the age of 9 years, few of the children in the sample had evidence of OME: only nine children had bilateral B tympanograms and 19 had a history of tubes bilaterally.

The developmental measures administered at Phase IX, and the methods of data analysis, were the same as those used at Phase VII. The means and standard deviations are presented in Table 6.8 and the results of the analysis in Table 6.9.

Given the findings obtained at Phase VII, it was anticipated that if any significant difference between groups were to be found at Phase IX, it would be for the measure of verbal expression. However, when the Bilateral B group and the Bilateral Tubes group were compared on each of the above measures, no significant differences between these groups were found. Similarly, when these groups were combined into a Bilateral B/Tubes group and compared with the Bilateral A group on each of the measures, again no significant differences were obtained, indicating that the children with evidence of OME at Phase IX did not differ significantly from those with no evidence of OME on any of the measures.

Finally, when the sums of squares for all remaining comparisons were pooled, a significant F test resulted for only one of the nine measures, that of speech articulation ($F=3.06$; $df=4, 742$; $p<0.05$). Separate *post hoc* comparisons revealed that none of the remaining differences between groups, on this measure, were significant at the $p \leq 0.01$ level.

Phase XI results

No attempt was made to examine the data obtained at Phase XI for developmental consequences. This decision was taken for two main reasons. Firstly, only 10 cases of bilateral B tympanograms were identified at this phase and no history was obtained or examination made for tympanostomy tubes. And secondly, the results obtained at previous phases suggested that no significant differences would be found. That is, at Phase VII, the combined Bilateral B/Tubes group had been found to differ significantly from the Bilateral A group on only one of the measures (verbal expression), while at Phase IX, no significant differences had been obtained between groups.

Longitudinal analysis

A limitation of the cross-sectional approach is that it enables comparisons between groups to be made at only a single point in time—in the present case, at a single age. The comparisons made on data collected at any one phase of the present

TABLE 6.8
Means and standard deviations for developmental measures at Phase IX

Group (at Phase IX)	*Intelligence*						*Verbal comprehension*		*Verbal expression*		*Speech articulation*		*Word reading*		*Behaviour problems**			
	Verbal		*Performance*		*Full scale*										*Parents*		*Teachers*	
	Mean	*SD*	*Mean*	*SD*	*Mean*	*SD*	*Mean*	*SD*	*Mean*	*SD*	*Mean*	*SD*	*Mean*	*SD*	*Mean*	*SD*	*Mean*	*SD*
Bilateral A	103.65	15.04	105.60	14.26	104.96	14.26	34.94	7.38	36.09	8.98	16.40	2.85	54.16	18.58	7.75	5.30	3.84	4.86
Bilateral B	108.67	14.57	105.67	17.76	108.17	16.53	34.33	11.81	38.83	9.91	16.80	1.92	60.33	19.60	5.33	2.25	4.17	5.15
Unilateral B	98.25	26.08	103.38	15.41	100.62	20.11	33.62	8.62	31.12	9.11	14.38	4.50	48.62	17.04	10.86	8.23	5.62	7.40
Bilateral Tubes	99.00	16.59	101.37	11.97	99.95	14.02	33.79	8.88	34.79	7.14	15.68	3.45	50.05	17.73	7.65	5.43	4.89	5.37
Unilateral Tube	92.00	21.21	98.38	16.97	94.62	20.28	31.88	8.44	30.75	15.58	13.38	5.40	46.88	19.01	10.62	4.93	2.62	2.50
Bilateral C	102.56	15.76	103.93	16.24	103.52	16.39	34.72	8.06	34.90	9.55	16.24	2.86	55.85	18.27	8.01	5.57	4.06	5.04
Unilateral C	103.03	15.66	105.88	14.38	104.73	15.20	35.67	7.69	35.26	8.99	16.08	3.19	51.26	20.12	8.78	5.87	4.57	5.27

*A higher score indicates more behaviour problems.

TABLE 6.9
Comparisons between means for developmental measures at Phase IX

Developmental measure	*Bilateral B* vs. *Bilateral Tubes*			*Average of Bilateral B and Bilateral Tubes* vs. *Bilateral A*			*All other comparisons (pooled sums of squares)*		
	F	*df*	*Sig.*	*F*	*df*	*Sig.*	*F*	*df*	*Sig.*
Intelligence									
Verbal	1.76	1, 742	*ns*	0.00	1, 742	*ns*	1.47	4, 742	*ns*
Performance	0.39	1, 742	*ns*	0.35	1, 742	*ns*	1.01	4, 742	*ns*
Full scale	1.36	1, 742	*ns*	0.06	1, 742	*ns*	1.42	4, 742	*ns*
Verbal comprehension	0.02	1, 742	*ns*	0.23	1, 742	*ns*	0.79	4, 742	*ns*
Verbal expression	0.89	1, 742	*ns*	0.11	1, 742	*ns*	1.58	4, 742	*ns*
Speech articulation	0.56	1, 727	*ns*	0.04	1, 727	*ns*	3.06	4, 742	*
Word reading	1.36	1, 742	*ns*	0.05	1, 742	*ns*	1.54	4, 742	*ns*
Behaviour problems									
Parent reports	0.78	1, 719	*ns*	0.90	1, 719	*ns*	1.82	4, 719	*ns*
Teacher reports	0.09	1, 737	*ns*	0.33	1, 737	*ns*	0.95	4, 737	*ns*

*$p<0.05$; *ns* = not significant.

study, therefore, were independent of those made on data collected at all other phases. From these comparisons, it is known only that there were significant differences between those children with and without evidence of OME on a single measure at Phase III, on four measures at Phase V and on a single measure at Phase VII. What is not known from these analyses is whether the effects of OME were transitory or long-lasting. To answer this question it was necessary to undertake a second, longitudinal analysis of the data.

The analysis reported below was designed to take advantage of the longitudinal data available on each child in the present study and to follow up an earlier analysis of the Phase V data reported by Silva *et al.* (1982). In that analysis, 47 children with bilateral OME at age 5 years were compared on various developmental measures with children who were otologically normal in both ears (N=357). 'OME' was defined as a Type B tympanogram plus otomicroscopically confirmed features of OME. 'Normal' was defined as a Type A tympanogram, also confirmed as normal by otomicroscopic examination. There were no significant differences between the groups in paternal socio-economic status, maternal verbal ability, maternal training in child development, or scores on a checklist of childhood experiences (Silva and Fergusson 1976), suggesting that the two groups were similar in background characteristics. At age 5 the bilateral OME group had significantly poorer hearing, a lower mean IQ, poorer speech articulation and verbal comprehension ability, and gained lower scores on a motor performance test. The children with bilateral OME also had significantly more behaviour problems.

Comparison groups

The two groups compared in this analysis were those with bilateral OME at age 5 (bilateral Type B tympanogram, and effusion confirmed by microscopic examination) and those who were otologically normal (bilateral Type A tympanogram, no effusion on microscopic examination and no previous tympanostomy tubes inserted). The sample followed longitudinally consisted of from 39 to 44 of the original 47 children who had bilateral OME at age 5, and from 297 to 323 of the original 357 children who had been otologically normal at that age. Those of the original sample not included were either lost to follow-up because of failure to co-operate, because complete assessments were not carried out for every assessment phase, or because they were not available for assessment as they had moved away from Dunedin. Any discrepancies between the frequencies reported in this section and those reported in Chapter 4 are due to minor differences in the assignment of subjects to groups. These differences were not expected to affect the outcome of the analysis reported here.

It will be recalled that subjects who were identified as having OME at age 5 were referred to Dunedin Hospital for further otological assessment. When a child met the criteria for surgical treatment, tympanostomy tubes were inserted. Of the 47 children with bilateral OME at age 5, 22 had tubes inserted. These are likely to have been those with more severe OME.

As noted earlier, the parents of children in the bilateral OME and the otologically normal groups did not differ significantly in terms of paternal socio-

TABLE 6.10
Mean Z scores* for Bilateral OME and Normal groups: longitudinal results

	Intelligence		*Verbal comprehension*		*Verbal expression*		*Speech*		*Word reading*		*Behaviour problems†* *Parents*		*Behaviour problems†* *Teachers*	
	OME (N=41)	*Normal (N=311)*	*OME (N=40)*	*Normal (N=307)*	*OME (N=40)*	*Normal (N=307)*	*OME (N=39)*	*Normal (N=297)*	*OME (N=44)*	*Normal (N=323)*	*OME (N=39)*	*Normal (N=298)*	*OME (N=39)*	*Normal (N=311)*
Age														
3 years	−0.11	0.04	−0.21	0.09	−0.20	0.08	—	—	—	—	—	—	—	—
5 years	−0.29	0.11	−0.36	0.08	−0.10	0.03	−0.41	0.04	—	—	0.34	−0.02	0.26	−0.08
7 years	0.03	0.10	0.04	0.06	−0.30	0.08	−0.34	0.09	−0.30	0.10	0.19	−0.10	0.49	−0.07
9 years	0.01	0.01	−0.14	0.01	−0.08	0.09	−0.46	0.12	−0.21	0.07	0.13	−0.09	0.25	−0.08
11 years	−0.03	0.05	—	—	—	—	—	—	−0.25	0.06	−0.01	−0.08	0.24	−0.03
F ratio‡	1.63		4.07		4.77		13.47		5.24		3.38		9.38	
Significance	0.202		0.044		0.030		0.001		0.023		0.067		0.002	

*Z scores have a mean of 0 and a standard deviation of 1.
†Higher scores indicate more behaviour problems.
‡F ratio for comparison of combined means.

TABLE 6.11
Means and standard deviations of three-frequency average hearing threshold levels by age

Age	*Bilateral OME group*			*Normal group*			*t test*	*Sig.*
	N	*Mean*	*SD*	*N*	*Mean*	*SD*		
5 years	46	20.1	9.3	351	4.6	3.8	20.8	p<0.001
7 years	44	12.8	5.2	330	10.0	4.5	3.7	p<0.001
9 years	39	11.6	5.6	306	8.7	4.1	4.0	p<0.001
11 years	40	11.5	5.8	294	7.9	4.9	4.2	p<0.001

economic status, maternal ability or maternal training in child development, and the children did not differ significantly in previous childhood experiences. They did differ significantly in mean binaural hearing at age 5, with the bilateral OME group having a mean three-frequency average (500, 1000 and 2000Hz) hearing level of 20.2dB (SD 10.18) compared with 4.6dB (SD 4.40) for the otologically normal group (Silva et al. *1982)*.

Results

The developmental measures used in this analysis were fully described in Chapter 2 (p. 48–49) and with the exception of those obtained at Phase XI, have been summarized above. Those obtained at Phase XI were as follows.

1. Intelligence—WISC: Full Scale.
2. Reading—Burt Word Reading Test.
3. Behaviour problems—Rutter Child Scales A (parents) and B (teachers).

All the scores, with the exception of the audiological results, were converted to Z scores with a mean of 0 and a standard deviation of 1. This was done to allow for a direct comparison of all measures.

The SPSS-X Manova procedure (SPSS Inc. 1983), incorporating a repeated measures design, was used to analyse the results. This procedure begins by looking for a group×time effect, that is, it tests whether the profiles of the means over time are parallel, or if there is an interaction between variables. If the interaction effect is not statistically significant, indicating that the profiles are parallel, the procedure tests the null hypothesis that there are no differences between the groups. There were no significant group×time effects for any of the analyses reported below, so the means of each of the comparison groups were combined and the groups compared. The combined means, F ratios and significance levels for each of the comparisons are presented in Table 6.10.

SEX DIFFERENCES

Of the 47 children with bilateral OME at age 5, 27 were boys and 20 were girls. In the comparison (otologically normal) group of 357 children, 170 were boys and 187 were girls. The sex difference was not statistically significant ($p>0.05$), so all results are reported for combined sexes.

HEARING LOSS AT AGES 5, 7, 9 AND 11 YEARS

The means and standard deviations of the three-frequency average threshold levels of the two groups are set out in Table 6.11. These were compared at each age, using

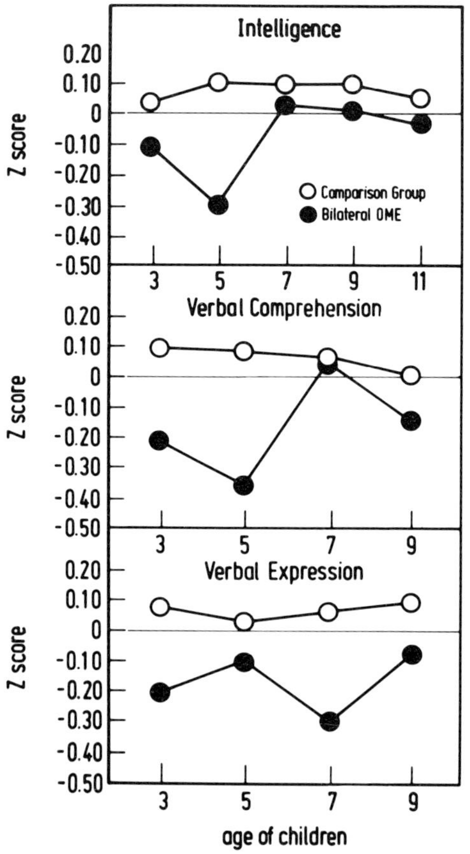

Fig. 6.1. Intelligence and language test results.

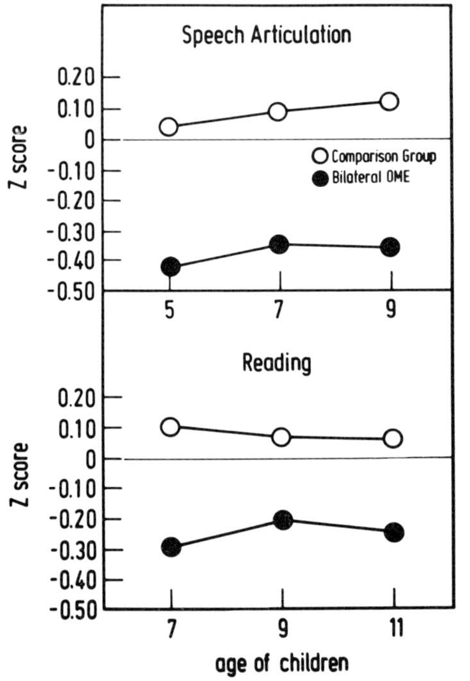

Fig. 6.2. Speech articulation and reading test results.

Student's t test. All differences were significant ($p<0.001$). The largest difference in means was at age 5; the difference at subsequent ages was much smaller.

INTELLIGENCE

The means of the intelligence test Z scores are set out in Table 6.10 and the results are depicted in Figure 6.1. The F ratio indicated that there was no significant difference between the combined means of the OME and Normal groups ($p>0.05$). While there was a relatively large difference in mean Z scores at age 5, differences at other ages were minor.

LANGUAGE DEVELOPMENT

The means for the verbal comprehension and verbal expression Z scores are also set out in Table 6.10 and the results depicted in Figure 6.1. The F ratios indicated that for both types of language measure there was a significant difference between the combined means for the two groups ($p<0.05$), with the bilateral OME group having the lower mean score. Figure 6.1 shows that there were larger differences

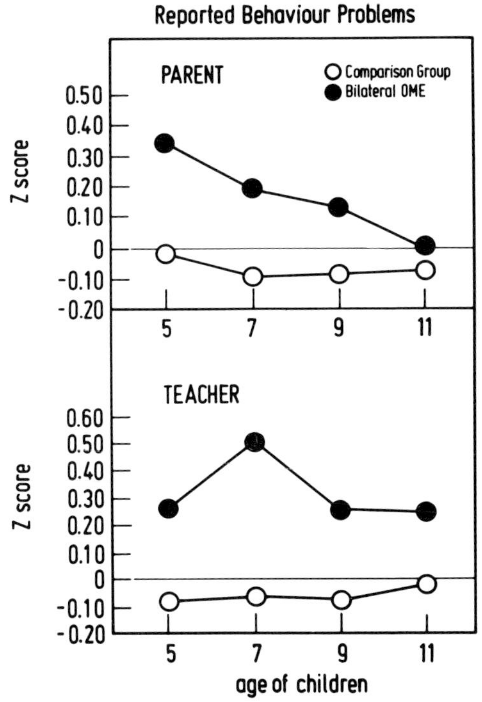

Fig. 6.3. Reported behaviour problems.

between the language comprehension test means at ages 3 and 5 than at 7 and 9. The figure also shows that the differences in expressive language mean scores were largest at ages 3 and 7, and smaller at ages 5 and 9.

SPEECH

The means of the speech test Z score results are set out in Table 6.10 and depicted in Figure 6.2. The F ratio indicated that the two groups were significantly different ($p<0.001$). The differences between the groups at ages 5, 7 and 9 remained consistently large.

READING

The means of the reading test Z scores are also set out in Table 6.10 and depicted in Figure 6.2. The F ratio indicated that the combined means for the two groups were significantly different ($p<0.05$). The difference between the means was largest at age 7 but was also relatively large at ages 9 and 11.

BEHAVIOUR PROBLEMS

The means of the Rutter Parents' and Teachers' Scales Z scores are set out in Table 6.10 and depicted in Figure 6.3. The F ratio obtained from analysis of the Parents' Scale results showed no significant group difference between the combined means

($p>0.05$). While differences between the groups were relatively large at ages 5 and 7, these narrowed by ages 9 and 11.

Analysis of the Teachers' Scale results demonstrated a significant group difference between the combined means ($p<0.01$), with the bilateral OME group gaining the highest behaviour problem scores. There were relatively large differences in teacher-reported behaviour problem scores at each age with the largest difference being found at age 7.

Discussion

An investigation was undertaken into the developmental consequences of hearing loss secondary to OME in the Dunedin sample. Two approaches were taken in this investigation. The first involved a cross-sectional analysis of data collected at Phases III, V, VII and IX of the study, in which children with and without evidence of OME at each phase were compared on a variety of developmental measures. In addition, children with MEP more negative than $-100mmH_2O$ were compared with tympanometrically normal children on the same measures.

The second approach involved a longitudinal follow-up of children who at Phase V had evidence of OME. The performance of these children on various developmental measures collected over the five phases of the study was compared with the performance over the same period of a group of children who at Phase V were otologically normal.

Cross-sectional analysis

The cross-sectional analysis of the data for each phase began with the comparison of those children with type B tympanograms bilaterally and those with tympanostomy tubes bilaterally. At only Phase VII were significant differences found between these two groups on any of the developmental measures. These were the measures of verbal comprehension and verbal expression, the level of significance being $p<0.05$ in each case. It was therefore reasonable to combine these two groups in all but the above two instances, for the purpose of comparison with the Bilateral A group. By this means the size of the group with the evidence of OME at each phase was increased, thereby adding to the reliability of the findings. This combined group will be referred to as the Bilateral OME group in the following discussion.

From the analysis of the data it was found that the Bilateral OME group differed significantly from the Bilateral A (normal) group on several of the developmental measures administered. These were *intelligence*, at age 5; *verbal comprehension*, at ages 3 and 5; *verbal expression*, at ages 3, 5, and 7 (Bilateral Tubes group only); and *behaviour problems*, as reported by teachers, at age 5. The mean scores, differences between means, and significance levels for these comparisons are summarized in Table 6.12. The two groups were found not to differ significantly on any of the measures administered at age 9, or at any age on the measures of speech articulation, reading, and behaviour problems reported by parents.

These findings suggest that OME affected the development of those children for whom the disease occurred bilaterally before the age of 5 years. At 7 years there

TABLE 6.12
Significant comparisons from the cross-sectional analysis at Phases III and V

Developmental measure	*Means* Combined Bilateral OME/ Tubes group*	*Normal group*	*Difference between means*	*Sig.*
Phase III				
Verbal comprehension	31.72	35.59	−3.87	p<0.01
Verbal expression	34.08	36.46	−2.38	p<0.05
Phase V				
Intelligence	99.22	106.91	−7.69	p<0.01
Verbal comprehension	49.34	51.18	−1.84	p<0.01
Verbal expression	48.08	50.26	−2.18	p<0.05
Behaviour problems[1]	4.36	3.14	1.22	p<0.05
Phase VII				
Verbal expression[2]	26.00	30.14	−4.14	p<0.05

*Means for the two groups averaged.
[1]Teachers' reports.
[2]Bilateral Tubes group only.

was only one significant effect for this group, while at 9 years there were no significant effects.

The findings further suggest that performance on the measure of intelligence was not affected until age 5, at which time the mean score was lower than that for the otologically normal group by almost eight IQ points. This difference was highly significant ($p<0.01$). Verbal skills, on the other hand, seemed to be affected earlier on, at age 3, with the mean score on the measure of verbal comprehension being almost four points lower than for the tympanometrically normal children, and that for the measure of verbal expression being down by nearly two-and-a-half points. The first of these differences was highly significant ($p<0.01$) while the second was significant at the $p\leq0.05$ level. The effect on verbal skills was also apparent at 5 years, but the magnitude of the deficit was less than at age 3 for both measures. These findings support recent research reported by Jerger *et al.* (1983) and Teele *et al.* (1984) who obtained similar effects with children aged from 2 to 5 years.

It is of interest that the Bilateral OME group at age 7 also scored significantly lower on the measure of verbal expression than the Bilateral A group. While only some of the children in this group at age 7 had been in it at age 5 also, this would suggest that the effect on verbal expression may be one of the more persistent developmental consequences of the disease. Evidence which supports this hypothesis is discussed later in this chapter.

The final significant effect obtained from this cross-sectional analysis was that the bilateral OME group at age 5 had significantly more behaviour problems, as observed by teachers, than the otologically normal children. The difference between the group means was a little over one point, at a significance level of $p<0.05$. This result supports an earlier suggestion by Gottlieb *et al.* (1979) of an association between OME and behaviour problems.

When the data were examined for other differences between groups, it was found, using a relatively conservative criterion ($p<0.01$), that none was significant. That is, the Unilateral B, Unilateral Tubes, Bilateral C and Unilateral C groups did not differ significantly from the Bilateral A group, or from each other, on any of the developmental measures administered. No evidence was found, therefore, of an association between unilateral OME, as evidenced by a type B tympanogram, and measures of intelligence, verbal skills or behaviour problems. Similarly, no evidence was found of an association between middle-ear pressure more negative than $-100mmH_2O$, either bilaterally or unilaterally, and any of the above developmental measures.

The effect of age at onset of OME on the developmental consequences of the disease was investigated during the analysis of the Phase VII data. This involved dividing the Bilateral B and Bilateral Tubes groups at Phase VII into those first identified at age 5 and those first identified at age 7. These groups were then compared on the developmental measures administered at Phase VII and it was found that the two did not differ significantly on any of these.

Longitudinal analysis

While there was a large difference between the mean binaural hearing levels of the bilateral OME and normal groups at age 5 (difference 15.6dB HTL), this was much less at ages 7 (2.8dB HTL), 9 (2.9dB HTL) and 11 (3.6dB HTL). This may reflect the effects of otological intervention in the more severe cases. Although the differences remained statistically significant in the later years, they were probably not large enough to be of clinical significance and would probably not have been marked enough from age 7 onwards to contribute to learning or other problems at those ages. As emphasized in the earlier report (Silva *et al.* 1982), it is possible that the hearing problems experienced by the children at age 5 could have contributed to less than optimal test performance at that time. This, however, is unlikely to have been the case from age 7 onwards.

The results from the intelligence tests showed a relatively large difference between the OME and Normal groups at age 5 but not at age 3 or at ages 7 to 9, and the overall difference between the combined means was not statistically significant. Had the results from the intelligence testing been the only ones reported, it would have been reasonable to suggest that the effects of bilateral OME are transitory. Also, had these results alone been reported, they would have given support to the view that the bilateral OME at age 5 was of recent onset, as the difference in results at age 3 was relatively small. Such results, had they been considered on their own, may also have suggested that the large difference between the intelligence test results at age 5 simply reflected the hearing loss experienced by the 5-year-old children at the time of testing. The results from the other measures, however, were somewhat different and lend no support to the above interpretations.

The language comprehension and language expression results showed that the difference between the combined means for the two groups was statistically significant. Also, at age 3 the bilateral OME group gained considerably lower scores than the comparison group on these measures. This finding suggests that the bilateral OME that had been identified at age 5 could have been present well before age 3 and could have had such a marked effect on hearing as to interfere with normal language development before that age. This hypothesis is important; if it were to gain more support, it could indicate the need to target efforts to identify and treat the problem well before children reach their third birthday. As has been demonstrated elsewhere (Fundudis *et al.* 1979, Reichman and Healey 1983, Silva *et al.* 1983), early language development is important since children with early language delay are a high risk group for later low intelligence, lower than average reading attainment and behavioural problems.

There was a lack of consistency in the language comprehension and expression results from age 5 onwards. At age 5 there was a relatively large difference in language comprehension scores between the groups, but at age 7 the difference was relatively small. The opposite pattern was seen with the expressive language results where there was a relatively large difference between the groups at age 7 but not at age 5. By age 9, the size of the difference between the groups was similar for both language measures. It was of interest that the language comprehension results showed a similar pattern to the intelligence test results.

The differences between the groups on the speech tests were consistently large over the three ages at which speech articulation was assessed (5, 7 and 9 years). Approximately 0.4 of a Z score separated the means at each age. Clearly, the bilateral OME group had consistently poorer speech articulation at each age and there was no sign of improvement by age 9. Likewise, those in the bilateral OME group gained consistently and significantly lower reading test scores than the comparison group from ages 7 to 11. While the difference was slightly greater at age 7, there was relatively little change in the difference between ages 9 and 11.

The results from the two behaviour problems measures were different. For parent-reported behaviour problems, there was a relatively large difference at age 5 but this decreased steadily to age 11. Over the four ages included in this analysis, the difference between the groups was not statistically significant. This suggests that parent-reported behaviour problems associated with OME at age 5 may be somewhat transitory. In contrast to these results, however, was the finding that the differences between the groups in teacher-reported behaviour problems were of a similar magnitude at ages 5, 9 and 11. Interestingly, there was a larger difference reported at age 7, the age by which the majority of children begin to make fairly rapid progress in reading. It should be noted that different results from the parent and teacher scales are not unexpected as the correlation between them is low (Rutter *et al.* 1970, McGee *et al.* 1983).

In the earlier study conducted on only the Phase V data (Silva *et al.* 1982), the question was raised about the later progress and adjustment of those children in the sample who experienced bilateral OME at age 5. This longitudinal analysis has shown that the intelligence differences were not sustained, although there was an overall significant difference in language development from ages 3 to 9. Both speech articulation and reading scores were significantly and consistently depressed in the bilateral OME group compared with those in the comparison group. Finally, teacher-reported but not parent-reported behaviour problems were significantly and consistently more prevalent in those who had bilateral OME. Therefore, in contrast to the cross-sectional results reported above, these results suggest that children who experience bilateral OME at the age of 5 and probably earlier, tend to remain significantly disadvantaged in some important aspects of their development through the mid-childhood years.

Conclusions

In the cross-sectional analysis, the developmental consequences of OME and MEP more negative than $-100mmH_2O$ were examined at each phase separately. From this approach, it was found that those children with evidence of bilateral OME at 5 years of age were significantly disadvantaged with regard to several aspects of their development. Those with bilateral OME at age 7 were affected in only one area, verbal expression, while 9-year-olds were unaffected by the disorder. No comparisons were made at age 11. No significant effects were obtained at any phase for those children with MEP more negative than $-100mmH_2O$.

In the longitudinal analysis, all of the 5-year-olds with bilateral OME were traced in their development from age 3 until age 11. From this approach, it was found that some of the disadvantages identified at 5 years persisted into the mid-childhood years. There seems to be good evidence from this analysis that early onset bilateral OME has long-lasting consequences with respect to language development, speech articulation, reading and teacher-reported behaviour problems.

Since this is the first longitudinal study of the long-term development of children with OME to be reported, it is essential that further longitudinal research be conducted to replicate the present findings and to resolve this long-standing and controversial issue. In the meantime, the present results give further support to current efforts toward the early identification and treatment of bilateral OME. They suggest that 5 years is too late an age to identify and deal with the problem, as children identified at that age are likely to perform significantly more poorly than others in a variety of areas, through the mid-childhood years. Some evidence emerged to suggest that even 3 years of age may be too late, although further research on the significance of bilateral OME for earlier child development is needed before such a conclusion can be supported with confidence.

It is appropriate, finally, to comment on the quality of the research reported in this chapter. Much of the criticism levelled at previous research was concerned with the sampling of subjects. Sample size and biased sampling procedures were of particular concern to critics. As explained in Chapter 2, the sample used in this study was drawn from an initial cohort of 1661 infants born in Dunedin, New Zealand, during a single 12 month period. The size of the sample at Phase V of the study was 917 children, declining to 803 at Phase XI. It has been acknowledged that the sample at Phase III was slightly biased in favour of subjects of higher socio-economic status, and was under-representative of Maori and other Polynesian children. The representativeness of the sample has been largely unaffected by the loss of subjects since Phase III. The sample, therefore, can be considered large in comparison to those used in most previous studies in this area and involved a cross-section of the population of children born in Dunedin. The sample cannot be taken to be representative of the overall New Zealand population of children.

Care has been taken in this study to avoid the methodological problems identified in much of the earlier research. The testing procedures were described in Chapter 2, the validity and reliability of the developmental measures have been documented elsewhere, as indicated in Chapter 2, and the procedures prescribed for these were adhered to. Finally, a conservative approach was taken in both the analysis and interpretation of results, so that charges of bias might be avoided. Consequently, the authors have confidence in the reliability and validity of the conclusions drawn above, with the proviso that replication studies are needed, especially with children under the age of 3 years.

7
OTOLOGICAL OBSERVATIONS

Introduction
Although international prevalence rates for OME are available to some degree (see Chapter 1, pp. 8–9), little epidemiological information exists as to the prevalence of more significant problems such as chronic perforation of the tympanic membrane or cholesteatoma. It is generally recognized that chronic perforation of the pars tensa is common in such populations as rural New Zealand Maori, Australian Aborigines, Eskimos, North American Indians and Vietnamese (Clements and Joseph 1981, Bluestone and Klein 1983, Sunderman and Dyer 1984). It is also recognized that chronic perforation of the tympanic membrane is relatively less common in people of African descent. In Europeans, chronic tympanic membrane perforation is thought to be associated with low socio-economic status.

By contrast, epidemiological data on cholesteatoma is singularly lacking. Cholesteatoma is probably the most serious commonly encountered ear disease, with its potential for causing deafness and offensive ear discharge, or even serious intracranial complications such as meningitis or brain abcess.

As shown in Chapter 4 (pp. 84–88), OME is an extremely common problem in children. Surgical procedures directed toward correction of this problem undoubtedly are the most commonly performed in the developed world—in the United States, over one million operations to treat OME are carried out per annum (Black 1984, Stickler 1984). At a cost per operation exceeding $US1000, OME has a significant economic impact.

Against this background, it seemed reasonable to attempt to evaluate the epiodemiology of chronic tympanic membrane perforation and cholesteatoma. The otological complications of surgical therapy for OME were also considered worthy of study.

Methods
The otological observations reported in this chapter were conducted primarily at Phases V, VII, IX and XI of the study. In addition a subsample of the children was examined at the age of 6 years (*i.e.* Phase VI).

Phase V
The children were examined by a trained medical officer. All children showing an otological abnormality or a B tympanogram were reviewed at weekly sessions by the principal investigator (IAS), so that only a few days elapsed between the first and second otological examinations. Children considered to have a significant otological abnormality at the second examination were then referred to the Dunedin Hospital Otolaryngology Service where they were followed up by the principal investigator and managed on purely clinical grounds. Management included antibiotic and decongestant therapy, tympanostomy tubes where considered indicated, and also associated surgical measures such as adenotonsillectomy

and antral lavage. When tympanostomy tubes were inserted, these were of the Teflon collar button pattern, placed inferiorly or postero-inferiorly in the tympanic membranes. Clinical follow-up was according to the routine of the clinic, with a maximum of six months between follow-up appointments. The parents were instructed to contact the clinic immediately in the event of problems such as pain, purulent ear discharge or recurrent deafness.

Phase VI

At Phase VI a total of 485 children were assessed, comprising a random subsample of those assessed at Phase V, those who had type C tympanograms at Phase V, and a group of 123 children who had been missed from the sample at Phase V (Stewart 1981).

As at Phase V, children showing otological abnormalities or type B tympanograms were seen by the principal investigator at weekly clinics and referred to the hospital services as required.

Phases VII, IX and XI

At phases VII, IX and XI, the entire sample was examined by a trained medical officer and once again weekly round-up clinics were held with consequent referral to the principal investigator at the hospital if a significant otological abnormality was noted and the child was not already under the care of the hospital clinic. A minimal number of children were referred at Phase XI.

Treatment

Between phases V and XI of the study, 195 children were managed by the Dunedin Hospital Otolarngyology Service. Information was available for the very small numbers of children treated privately. Of 142 children detected as having middle-ear effusion between Phases V and VII of the study the outcome was known to the principal investigator in 139 cases. One child was known to have been treated with tympanostomy tubes elsewhere, and in two children (both with unilateral problems) the outcome was unknown.

It was policy to follow up all children with evidence of a problem (such as OME), until at least six months after resolution of the problem. Children with potentially serious problems were followed indefinitely. Those with deep retraction pockets requiring surgical reconstruction were followed for five years following surgery. Those requiring simple drum repair were followed for two years postoperatively. Children with lesser tympanic membrane abnormalities were followed until it was apparent that the abnormality was stable and no dangers to hearing or health remained.

Results

Results are reported as categorized on the study findings up to Phase IX, with the addition of data available from the Otolaryngology Service over the following two years. The commonest otological condition diagnosed was OME. Because of the nature of this condition, with its tendency to remission and relapse, description is difficult. The descriptive problem is increased by the fact that intervention took place. Medical and surgical intervention requires a double-blind control design over a large sample before any conclusions can be drawn as to the effects of therapy.

Such observations are not appropriate to this sample, which is simply described, although some pointers toward factors requiring study in a controlled fashion may be obtained from this descriptive study. There is a gradation in the severity of OME and the following categorization reflects this variation in severity, with division of the OME cases into the following arbitrary groups.

1. Transient OME—unilateral and bilateral. These children had OME diagnosed microscopically on one or two occasions in the course of the evaluation. On no occasion did the OME persist for longer than three months, or require surgical therapy.
2. Persistent OME—unilateral or bilateral, not requiring surgical intervention in the form of tympanostomy tubes. These children had no more than two episodes of OME, neither greater than three months duration. The severity of the symptoms was considered insufficient to warrant surgical intervention.
3. Unilateral Tube. These children had unilateral OME which was adjudged of sufficient severity to warrant the insertion of a tympanostomy tube, on the grounds of pain, recurrent otitis media or clinical concern about the appearance of the tympanic membrane.
4. Bilateral Tubes. These children had tympanostomy tubes inserted in both ears on one occasion for the treatment of OME which had persisted for longer than three months and was giving rise to clinical concern, on such grounds as hearing loss, educational or behavioural problems, pain, recurrent otitis or clinical concern at the appearances of the tympanic membranes.
5. Repeated Tubes. These children had tympanostomy tubes inserted in both ears on more than one occasion, the grounds being similar to the previous group and the problem relapsing upon extrusion of the tympanostomy tube.

The number of children assigned to each of the above groups is noted in Table 7.1.

Complications of tympanostomy tubes

The following complications were experienced by the 101 children having tympanostomy tubes inserted into 184 ears. Purulent discharge from the ear, or associated formation of granulation tissue in relation to the tubes, was experienced in 21 cases. All these local infections responded to medical treatment and in no case was it necessary to remove the tympanostomy tube.

Perforation of the tympanic membrane occurred in 16 ears following extrusion of the tympanostomy tube. 11 of these perforations healed spontaneously and five required surgical measures for closure. Of these five, two required formal myringoplasty and three healed following minor outpatient procedures to stimulate healing.

Retraction pockets

Although a small atrophic scar is a common consequence of a tympanostomy tube (see below), such a scar in the presence of ongoing middle-ear problems may result in a retraction pocket. Atrophic scars may also result from acute otitis media,

TABLE 7.1
Categorization of the sample

*Group**	*f*	%
Transient OME	118	12.3
Persistent OME	23	2.4
Unilateral Tube	18	1.9
Bilateral Tubes	70	7.3
Repeated Tubes	13	1.4
Neither OME nor tube	720	74.7
Total sample	962	100.0

*See text for definition of groups.

especially when associated with perforation. When retraction pockets arise in the postero-superior quadrant of the tympanic membrane, these are of particular significance, as they may retract onto the incus and stapes head, or even more deeply into the facial recess, where a cholesteatoma may arise if there is retention of keratin. Additionally, adhesion of the retraction pocket to the long process of the incus and stapes head may produce destruction of these ossicles.

Twelve postero-superior retraction pockets were noted in the sample, eight of these in cases where tympanostomy tubes had previously been inserted. Eight of the retraction pockets were regarded as insignificant and there was no evidence of either progression or incus destruction on long-term observation. Four of the retraction pockets, all from ears previously having tympanostomy tubes, were deep and were either associated with keratin retention or incus erosion. All of these ears were reconstructed surgically.

Perforation
It is noteworthy that no spontaneously occurring chronic perforation arose in the sample. Although perforation of the pars tensa of the tympanic membrane was noted in cases of acute otitis media, all such perforations healed spontaneously. The only cause of chronic perforation in the sample, therefore, was a previous tympanostomy tube.

Cholesteatoma and problems in the attic region
Unfortunately no system of recording the lesser degrees of attic retraction (such as that described by Tos and Poulsen 1980) was instituted when the study was commenced. One deep, self-cleansing attic retraction pocket was noted. Two attic cholesteatomas were observed in the sample. One of these occurred in an 8-year-old child who had previously required bilateral tympanostomy tubes and who continued to require bilateral tubes following surgical treatment of the cholesteatoma. Unfortunately this child suffered from extremely narrow external auditory meati with associated keratin retention and otitis externa; consequently adequate documentation of attic findings prior to the development of the cholesteatoma was not available. The second cholesteatoma presented as granulation tissue coming through the outer attic wall in a 12-year-old child. This child had experienced transient unilateral OME in the same ear at the age of 5 years, but no attic problem

TABLE 7.2
Tympanic membrane sequelae of children's ears (N=1508) at age 9 years

Group	*Normal* %	*Hyaline scar* %	*Calcified scar* %	*N*
Previous tube	18	21	61	142
Documented OME, no tube	63	33	4	174
Never documented OME	68	30	2	1192

had been noted at that time. This cholesteatoma may conceivably have been primary, as it did not link directly with the pars flaccida.

Bilateral tympanostomy tubes
The 13 children who required bilateral tympanostomy tubes on more than one occasion experienced more than average complications. At the age of 13 years, five of these children had satisfactory ears, two still had tubes in the tympanic membranes, four had experienced perforations which closed spontaneously, one had required surgery for attic cholesteatoma and three had required surgery for deep marginal retraction pockets. A further two had shallow retraction pockets which did not require surgery.

Tympanic membrane sequelae
The tympanic membrane sequelae at age 9 years are listed in Table 7.2. The children have been divided into three groups: those who had previous tympanostomy tubes, those with previously documented OME but no tympanostomy tubes, and those who never had OME documented. It should be borne in mind that only those ears showing severe problems had tubes inserted. However, it is obvious that calcified scar tissue in the tympanic membrane and also atrophic scars in the tympanic membrane were very much a feature of those ears which had tubes inserted. It is also apparent that approximately 30 per cent of ears which had documented milder effusions, and of those which had no documented effusion, showed hyaline scar tissue in the tympanic membrane. This is of little practical consequence in terms of hearing but does imply that there have been previous inflammatory episodes sufficient to cause objective changes in the tympanic membrane.

In Phases VII and IX, scar tissue in the tympanic membranes was carefully documented. Although this is difficult to express quantitatively, there was little doubt on analysing the results qualitatively that scar tissue which had been documented as present at the age of 7 had disappeared or was diminished in some cases at the age of 9. This applied to both hyaline and calcified scar tissue.

Conclusions
There are several conclusions to be drawn. A salient feature is the complete lack of spontaneous chronic perforation in the sample. All 16 perforations occurred following insertion of tympanostomy tubes. On the other hand, all but three of these perforations closed spontaneously or following fairly minor outpatient

procedures. This gives a risk of chronic perforation of 1.6 per cent—rather less if multiple tube insertions are considered. It should be pointed out that the tube used was of the 'collar button' pattern. This is a large tube which probably has a relatively high risk of producing a chronic perforation.

The other tympanic membrane sequelae of atrophic and calcified scars do appear to be associated with tympanostomy tubes, although again it should be pointed out that the tympanostomy tubes were inserted in those ears which had the most severe problems. This observation is in keeping with those of Kilby *et al.* (1972) and Tos *et al.* (1983*a*).

There is little doubt that atrophic scars in the tympanic membrane are associated with tympanostomy tubes. It is of concern to determine whether postero-superior retraction pockets may be caused by tympanostomy tubes. Retrospectively, the placement of tympanostomy tubes in the postero-inferior quadrant of the drum may have been an aetiological factor in causing retraction pockets. Tympanostomy tubes placed in this situation not infrequently migrate to a postero-superior position prior to extrusion, so that an atrophic scar occurs in this position. In the presence of continuing negative middle-ear pressure and/or effusion, the stage may be set for development of a retraction pocket.*

*The reader's attention is drawn to the results of a follow-up examination of the tympanic membranes of the sample, conducted at Phase XV of the Dunedin Multidisciplinary Health and Development Study (Stewart *et al.* 1989), which complete much of the investigation reported here.

8
SUMMARY AND CONCLUSIONS

Identification and diagnosis

Four methods of identification and diagnosis were used in the present study: history, otoscopy, impedance audiometry and pure-tone audiometry.

Otological history

An otological history was obtained for each child by means of a questionnaire administered to the parents when the children were 3, 5, 7 and 9 years of age. At 3 years, 3.5 per cent of the children were believed by their parents to have hearing problems; at 5 years, 4.8 per cent had had a confirmed hearing problem at some time in the past; and at 7 years, 15.6 per cent had had a hearing loss confirmed in the previous two years, as had 6.6 per cent at 9 years. When the children were 5 years old, parents were questioned in detail regarding past hearing problems. At this age, 132 children had had a suspected hearing problem, of whom 77.1 per cent had seen a doctor and 40.2 per cent had had the problem confirmed. In 66.7 per cent of cases it was the child's mother who had first suspected the hearing problem.

At 3 years, 16.1 per cent of the children were reported to have had one or more ear infections in the preceding year. At Phase V, 41.7 per cent were reported to have had an ear infection in the past two years; this figure declined to 39.2 per cent at Phase VII and 24.8 per cent at Phase IX. A significant relationship between reported ear infections and reported hearing problems was obtained at each of the four ages at which a history was obtained.

When the children were aged 5, parents reported that 25.6 per cent had had 'sore ears' on one or more occasion in the past, while 10 per cent were reported to have had a pus discharge on one or more occasions. These symptoms of OM were found to be significantly related to reported hearing problems. Information was also obtained at this age concerning actions taken by parents when the children had ear infections, sore ears or pus discharge. For ear infections, 92 per cent were seen by the family doctor, with 99 per cent of these receiving medication. Nine children were referred for specialist care, with five receiving surgical treatment. For sore ears, 55.6 per cent were seen by the family doctor, and 95 per cent of these received medication; nine were referred for specialist care and four received surgical treatment. Notably, for 40.8 per cent of children with sore ears, no action was taken by parents. For pus discharge, 82.2 per cent were seen by the family doctor, with 80 per cent receiving medication. Nine were referred for specialist care and five were treated surgically. It was apparent from these findings that parents regarded ear infections and pus discharge more seriously than sore ears, even though all were associated with hearing problems.

The history of a further two disorders associated with hearing problems was obtained when the children were aged 5. No relationship was found between hearing problems and the frequency of blocked nose, while a highly significant relationship between hearing problems and tonsillitis was revealed. Ear infections, sore ears, pus discharge, blocked nose and tonsillitis were all investigated as risk factors associated with OME.

A history of ear operations was obtained when the children were 7 years of age and again when they were 9. At 7 years, 89 children were reported to have had ear operations in the previous two years, of whom 78.7 per cent had had tympanostomy tubes inserted bilaterally. 20 per cent had a tube inserted unilaterally. At 9 years, 33 children had had ear operations in the previous two years, with 57.6 per cent being for bilateral tube insertion and 24.2 per cent for unilateral insertion.

Sixty-three of the children had had tonsillectomies and 97 had had adenoidectomies by the age of 9 years.

Finally, the parents of nine children (1.0 per cent) considered their child had had an accident due to a hearing problem, while those of a further 12 children reported 'near misses'.

Otological examination

Otological examinations were conducted when the children were 5, 7 and 9 years of age. From these, prevalence rates for OME of 9.0 per cent at 5 years, 6.0 per cent at 7 years and 2.5 per cent at 9 years were obtained. These were slightly lower than for other recently reported epidemiological studies but since most of these used impedance audiometry rather than otoscopy, the above figures were considered conservative.

A detailed analysis of the content of the otological examinations was conducted and from this it was concluded that the signs which best discriminated abnormal (OME) from normal ears were an abnormal light reflex, microvascularization of the tympanic membrane, translucency of the membrane, and observable secretions in the tympanic cavity.

Impedance audiometry

Impedance audiometry was conducted at 5, 7, 9 and 11 years. Middle-ear pressure was recorded at all four ages, static compliance and tympanometric gradients at ages 5, 7 and 9, and ipsilateral accoustic reflexes at ages 7 and 9. The findings for each of these measures are summarized below.

1. Middle-ear pressure declined from a mean of $-120mmH_2O$ at 5 years to $-84mmH_2O$ at 11. The proportion of ears with no pressure peak fell from 8.7 per cent at age 5 to 1.6 per cent at age 11.
2. The majority of ears fell within the normal limits for static compliance (*i.e.* 0.3 to $1.5cm^3$). 14 per cent of ears exceeded these limits at age 5, 9 per cent at age 7, and 11 per cent at age 9.
3. The gradients of the tympanograms were calculated according to the method of Paradise and Smith (1979). The mean gradient was around 0.67 at age 5, 0.73 at age 7, and 0.98 at age 9.

Ipsilateral acoustic reflex testing was conducted when the children were aged 7 years and again at age 9. Due to an error in the testing procedure, reflex thresholds recorded with the conventional impedance meter were discarded from the data analysis. When tested with the automatic impedance meter at age 9, reflexes were found to be absent in 32 per cent of right ears and 25.3 per cent of left ears.

The classification of ears by tympanogram type was conducted at each age at which testing was carried out. Assignment into one of seven groups was made on the basis of the shape of the tympanogram, middle-ear pressure and static compliance. The seven groups were as follows.

A = Normal shape, middle-ear pressure and compliance.
A_S = Compliance below normal range (0.3–1.5cm^3).
A_D = Compliance above normal range (0.3–1.5cm^3).
C_1 = Middle-ear pressure more negative than –100mmH_2O.
C_2 = Middle-ear pressure more negative than –200mmH_2O.
B/C = Compliance rising as –400mmH_2O is approached but not peaking before –400mmH_2O.
B = Flat or flattish curve, no measurable MEP peak.

At the age of 5 years, 8.8 per cent of ears were type B, indicating OME. This figure declined to 6.1 per cent at age 7, followed by a sharp drop to 1.8 per cent at age 9 and 1.3 per cent at age 11. Ears with type C tympanograms, indicating middle-ear pressure more negative than –100mmH_2O, declined from 39.2 per cent at 5 years to 25.4 per cent at 11. Ears with type B/C tympanograms declined from 1.7 per cent at age 5 to 1.1 per cent at age 11. Type A (normal) ears increased from 50.3 per cent at age 5 to 72.0 per cent at 11.

Comparison of impedance audiometry and otological examination
The two principal methods of detecting OME that were used in this study, otoscopy and impedance audiometry, were examined for the degree of correspondence between them. From the data gathered at age 5, it was found that 47 per cent of ears judged normal on examination by the otologist were found to have abnormal middle-ear pressure, or abnormal compliance when tested with an impedance meter. With regard to the identification of OME, there was agreement between the two methods in 107 cases, or 54 per cent of those identified by the two methods combined.

Epidemiology and risk factors
From the review of research on the epidemiology and natural history of OME and on risk factors associated with this disease, several deficiencies were identified. These included a lack of information on the prevalence of OME in children over the age of 7 years and on the prevalence of the disease in children in New Zealand. Further, it was noted that existing evidence on risk factors was often equivocal and that the quality of epidemiological research in this area in general was not high.

Prevalence
Taking a type B tympanogram (including type B/C) as evidence of OME, the following prevalence rates for the present sample were obtained: at age 5 years, 10.5 per cent; at 7 years, 6.5 per cent; at 9 years, 3.0 per cent; and at 11 years, 2.4 per cent.

The rates at 5 and 7 years were comparable to those reported in the studies reviewed in Chapter 1, while the low rates obtained at 9 and 11 years confirmed the view generally held by clinicians that OME declines rapidly from around 6 or 7 years of age.

When those children with tympanostomy tubes present at the time of testing were included in the prevalence rates, these rose to 12.5 per cent at 5 years, 9.4 per cent at 7 years, 3.5 per cent at nine years, with no change at age 11.

Another approach taken to describe the prevalence of OME in the sample was to identify those children with the disease in one or both ears at the time of examination. At 5 years of age, 15.1 per cent of the children were affected, this prevalence declining to 9.5 per cent at age 7, around 4.3 per cent at age 9 and 3.5 per cent at age 11. At all of the above ages, however, fewer children had OME bilaterally than had it unilaterally. When the children with tympanostomy tubes in place at the time of examination were included in the above figures, 17.4 per cent were found to have evidence of OME in one or both ears at 5 years, 12.9 per cent at 7 years, 5.2 per cent at 9 years and 3.5 per cent at 11 years.

The prevalence of type C tympanograms in the sample declined from 39.2 per cent at 5 years to 36.2 per cent at age 7, 29.8 per cent at age 9 and 25.4 per cent at age 11. The contribution made by middle-ear pressure more negative than $-100mmH_2O$ to the overall rate of middle-ear pathology in the sample rose from 79 per cent at 5 years to 91 per cent at 11 years.

Despite a steady decline in middle-ear pathology over the six years of the study, at age 11 years 28 per cent of ears were still affected in some way. As noted above, most in this group suffered from middle-ear pressure more negative than $-100mmH_2O$. Middle-ear pressure more negative than $-100mmH_2O$ was found not to be associated with significant audiological or developmental deficits.

Risk factors

For the investigation of risk factors the sample was divided into six longitudinal groups based on the study data and records of the Dunedin Hospital Otolaryngology Service, up to the age of 9 years. The findings revealed that the risk of OME declined beyond the age of 5 years, was greater in boys than in girls, and was greater in winter and spring than in summer or autumn. A history of ear infection, sore ears, pus discharge and nasal obstruction were all found to increase the risk of OME, as was a clinical diagnosis of nasal obstruction. All of the above findings were consistent with those of previous studies. At variance with the results of previous studies were the findings that the risk of OME is increased by tonsillitis and reduced by breast-feeding.

Factors found not to be associated with risk of OME were socio-economic status, respiratory allergy, perinatal characteristics (gestational age, birthweight, head circumference), parental smoking habits and attendance at group day-care or pre-school facilities. The evidence in relation to all of these factors remains equivocal.

A factor not previously investigated, and found in the present study to be associated with OME, is that of family adversity. It was found that two or more sources of adversity in a child's home environment increased the risk of OME.

Discussion

The prevalence rates presented above provide information in areas where this was lacking previously. Firstly, they confirm the view that the prevalence of OME declines rapidly from around 6 or 7 years of age. Secondly, they provide much needed information on the prevalence of OME in New Zealand children.

Regrettably, an important gap in knowledge of OME in children under the age of 5 years has not been filled by the present study. Given the belief, expressed in Chapter 6, that OME occurring during these early years may have long-term developmental consequences for the children concerned, it is important that priority be given to obtaining further information on the nature and prevalence of OME for this group.

The investigation of risk factors confirmed previous findings with regard to age, sex, season, several related disorders, and prevalence in right *vs.* left ears. The findings of the present study were inconsistent with previously reported results regarding breast-feeding and tonsillitis, while the evidence on socio-economic status, respiratory allergy, perinatal characteristics, parental smoking habits and exposure in group day-care remained equivocal. Using an index of family adversity, it was found that the presence of two or more sources of adversity in a child's home environment increased the risk of OME. This latter finding led to the conclusion that it may be more appropriate in future investigations to examine the cumulative effects of a variety of possible risk factors before rejecting any single factor such as socio-economic status.

Audiological characteristics

Hearing threshold levels

The mean hearing threshold levels (HTLs) for the full sample at 5 years of age were around 13dB at 500Hz, 8dB at 1000Hz, 0.5dB at 2000Hz and 1dB at 4000Hz. The average HTL over the three frequencies of 500, 1000 and 2000Hz was around 7dB at 5 years. HTLs were poorer at 7 years of age, when the means over the four frequencies were 16, 11, 6 and 8dB respectively, with a mean three-frequency average of 11dB. A very slight improvement in HTLs occurred at 9 and 11 years of age.

Middle-ear dysfunction

For the purpose of identifying the degree of hearing impairment associated with OME and related disorders, each ear was assigned to one of seven groups according to tympanogram type, as defined earlier in this chapter (p. 148). The mean HTLs at 500, 1000, 2000 and 4000Hz were calculated for both right and left ears at ages 5, 7, 9 and 11 years.

With few exceptions, the means for all seven groups fell within the limits of normal hearing (–10 to 26dB HTL) as defined by Green (1978). As expected, the mean HTLs for ears with evidence of OME (type B tympanogram) were significantly poorer than for normal ears (type A tympanogram) at all frequencies tested and at all four ages. In general, these were consistent with the average of 15 to 30dB HTL reported in previous studies. The configuration of HTLs over 500, 1000, 2000 and 4000Hz for the OME group at each age followed the pattern of previous studies, being relatively flat and with a slight peak at 2000Hz.

At none of the ages included in the study did the low compliance (type A_S tympanogram) or high compliance (type A_D tympanogram) groups differ significantly from the tympanometrically normal group (type A). Further, the configurations for these two groups followed a very similar pattern to those for normal ears, with the curves rising steadily between 500 and 2000Hz and then flattening out between 2000 and 4000Hz.

No consistent pattern of mean HTLs was apparent for the two negative middle-ear pressure groups (tympanogram types C_1 and C_2). It is noteworthy, however, that the mean HTLs for these groups were better than 20dB at all frequencies for all ages and were generally better than 15dB, particularly in the higher frequencies. The mean HTLs for the B/C tympanogram group were generally poorer than those for the type A tympanogram group but were generally better than 20dB.

It has been suggested that the average HTL across the three frequencies of 500, 1000 and 2000Hz provides a useful predictor of sensitivity for speech (Green 1978). This average is therefore useful when considering the developmental consequences of hearing loss secondary to OME.

For normal ears (type A tympanogram) the mean three-frequency average HTL was 4.3dB at 5 years, rising to 9.5dB at 7 years, then declining to 8.8dB at 9 years and 7.5dB at 11 years. This reflects the pattern of change in normal hearing described earlier. In contrast, for ears with OME, as indicated by a type B tympanogram, the means at 5 and 7 years were virtually identical at around 20dB HTL, rising to 23.7dB HTL at 9 years and 25.6dB HTL at 11 years. These means were all significantly poorer than those for the normal group (type A tympanogram), and although falling short of the mean hearing loss of 27.6dB HTL for ears with OME as stated by Bess (1983), exceeded the lower limit of mild hearing loss (15dB HTL) on Northern and Downs' (1978) scale of childhood hearing loss.

For ears with abnormally low (type A_S tympanogram) or abnormally high (type A_D tympanogram) compliance, the mean HTLs did not differ significantly from normal. When compared with normal ears, those with MEP more negative than –100mmH_2O but less negative than –200mmH_2O (type C_1 tympanogram) showed an inconsistent pattern of significant and non-significant differences. In contrast, those ears with MEP more negative than –200mmH_2O but less negative than –400mmH_2O (type C_2 tympanogram) were consistently poorer at all four ages, exceeding 10dB HTL at 7, 9 and 11 years. These findings confirmed the assertion by Bess (1983) that such losses could be expected to accompany negative middle-ear pressure, even in the absence of effusion. Finally, mean HTLs in ears with compliance rising but failing to peak before –400mmH_2O (type B/C tympanogram) increased from around 13dB HTL at 5 and 7 years to 18.7dB HTL at 9 years and 19.7dB HTL at 11 years.

Hearing in better ear

In order to obtain a better idea of the actual hearing loss suffered by children with OME or with middle-ear pressure more negative than –100mmH_2O, the hearing in the better ear of the children in the sample was examined. The groups used for this analysis were: Bilateral A, Bilateral B, Unilateral B, Bilateral Tubes, Unilateral Tube, Bilateral C, Unilateral C.

At each age, the mean HTLs of those children with bilateral B tympanograms were significantly poorer at each frequency than those of the children with bilateral A tympanograms. Generally, these means were poorer at 500Hz and 1000Hz, ranging from 18 to 23dB HTL, while at 2000Hz and 4000Hz they were often better than 15 dB HTL. The mean three-frequency average HTLs for this group were generally better than 20dB HTL. These means were all significantly poorer than those for the better ears of the type A group.

A trend which became apparent in the data was for the mean HTLs by frequency of the better ear of children with a unilateral B tympanogram to become poorer with age. This was most apparent when the mean three-frequency average HTLs were compared. These declined from 7.4dB at age 5 years to 12.7dB at age 7, 15dB at age 9 and 20.2dB at age 11.

At 5 years of age, the bilateral and unilateral tube groups did not differ significantly from each other or from the type A group at any frequency. At 7 and 9 years, however, the mean HTLs by frequency for the better ear of these children were significantly poorer than for the type A group. Nevertheless, they were better than 15dB HTL at all but 500Hz.

Finally, the mean HTLs of the better ear of those children with bilateral C tympanograms were significantly poorer than normal at 500, 1000 and 4000Hz but not at 2000Hz. In general, however, they were better than 15dB HTL and in the higher frequencies were better than 10dB HTL. The hearing in the better ear of children with a unilateral C tympanogram generally did not differ significantly from that of children in the type A group.

Developmental consequences

Perhaps the most important aspect of the present study was the investigation of the developmental consequences of OME. From the review of the literature on this subject, it was apparent that while many studies had been conducted over the previous two decades, much of this work had been severely criticized for inadequacies in the design of the research, in the analysis of the results and in the drawing of conclusions from these results. Two schools of thought on this research were identified: those who recognized the problem associated with it but who nevertheless believed that the weight of evidence indicated a causal link between OME and developmental problems, and those who believed that until its methodological inadequacies had been overcome, no firm conclusions could be drawn regarding this relationship. The literature review led to the conclusion that a fresh approach was needed to this question and that there was considerable support among the critics of past research for a longitudinal approach to be taken. Two approaches were adopted in investigating the developmental consequences of hearing loss secondary to OME in the Dunedin sample, the first cross-sectional and the second longitudinal.

Cross-sectional analysis

In this approach, children with and without evidence of OME at each phase were compared on a variety of developmental measures at the ages of 5, 7 and 9 years. Some measures administered when the children were 3 years old were included in this analysis. Similarly, children with middle-ear pressure more negative than $-100mmH_2O$ were compared with the tympanometrically normal children to determine if this disorder had developmental consequences.

This investigation revealed that children with evidence of bilateral OME at the time of testing (*i.e.* type B tympanogram or tubes) differed significantly from the tympanometrically normal group on measures of intelligence at 5 years, of verbal comprehension at ages 3 and 5, of verbal expression at ages 3, 5 and 7 (bilateral tubes only), and of teacher-reported behaviour problems at age 5. No significant differences were obtained for any of the measures administered at age 9, nor for measures of speech articulation, reading or parent-reported behaviour problems at any age. Given that only one significant effect was found at 7 years and none were found at 9, it was considered unnecessary to analyse the data collected at 11 years.

These findings suggested that OME had affected some aspects of the development of those children in whom the disease had occurred bilaterally before the age of 5 years. They were seen to support two recently reported studies which obtained similar effects with regard to intelligence and verbal skills for children aged from 2 to 5 years (Jerger *et al.* 1983, Teele *et al.* 1984). The significant difference in teacher-reported behaviour problems supported an earlier suggestion by Gottlieb *et al.* (1979) of an association between OME and behaviour problems.

With regard to those children having unilateral OME, a unilateral tube or middle-ear pressure more negative than $-100mmH_2O$, either bilaterally or unilaterally at the time of testing, no evidence was obtained to indicate that these conditions had any significant effect on intelligence, verbal skills or behaviour at any of the ages concerned.

Longitudinal approach

Since the above investigation involved separate and independent analyses at each of three ages, it was considered desirable to examine the data for the effect of OME over time. In this approach an earlier analysis of the data obtained when the children were 5 years of age (Silva *et al.* 1982) was followed up longitudinally. This approach involved taking those children with bilateral OME at 5 years (N=47) and following their development to age 11, contrasting this with the development of those children who were otologically normal in both ears at age 5 (N=355). A repeated measures design was used to analyse the data. The results of this analysis indicated that while a significant difference in intelligence scores between these two groups, identified at 5 years of age, was not sustained, disadvantages with respect to language development, speech articulation, reading and teacher-reported behaviour problems did persist into the mid-childhood years of those children who had had bilateral OME at age 5.

Because this is the first longitudinal study of the long-term development of children with OME to be reported, it is essential that further longitudinal research be conducted to replicate this finding and to clarify this longstanding and controversial issue. Such research should focus on younger children, preferably younger than 3 years. In the meantime, the present results give further support to current efforts toward the early identification and treatment of bilateral OME. There was some suggestion in these results that identification at age 5 may be too late to avoid the developmental consequences identified in this study. A need for further research on this question is indicated.

Otological observations

In comparison to OME, relatively little epidemiological information exists regarding the more significant problems of chronic perforation of the tympanic membrane and cholesteatoma. It was considered, therefore, that the epidemiology of these two problems should be evaluated. Further, given the high prevalence rates for OME found in this and other studies, it was considered that the otological complications of surgical therapy for OME should be evaluated also.

Since those children in the study who were considered to have significant otological abnormalities were referred to the Dunedin Hospital Otolaryngology Service, the record of their treatment was available for the proposed evaluations. A total of 195 children from the study were managed by the Otolaryngology Service.

On the basis of the study data up to Phase IX and the records of the Otolaryngology Service, 962 children were categorized as follows: transient OME (12.3 per cent), persistent OME (2.4 per cent), unilateral tube on one occasion (1.9 per cent), bilateral tubes on one occasion (7.3 per cent), bilateral tubes on more than one occasion (1.4 per cent), and neither OME nor tubes (74.7 per cent).

Of 101 children having tympanostomy tubes inserted into their ears, 21 experienced purulent discharge or the formation of granulation tissue in relation to the tubes. Perforation of the tympanic membrane occurred in 16 ears following extrusion of the tympanostomy tube.

Twelve postero-superior retraction pockets were noted in the sample, eight in cases where tympanostomy tubes had previously been inserted. There were no examples of spontaneously occurring chronic perforations. Therefore, the only cause of chronic perforation was a previous tympanostomy tube.

Two attic cholesteatomas were observed in the sample.

Of the 13 children who required bilateral tympanostomy tubes on more than one occasion, five had satisfactory ears at the age of 13; two still had tubes in the tympanic membrane; four had experienced perforations which closed spontaneously; one required surgery for attic cholesteatoma; three required surgery for deep marginal retraction pockets; and two had shallow retraction pockets which did not require surgery.

Calcified scar tissue and atrophic scars in the tympanic membrance were observed at age 9 years to be a common feature of those ears which earlier had had tympanostomy tubes inserted.

From the above findings it was concluded that the risk of chronic perforation following extrusion of a tympanostomy tube was 1.6 per cent, or rather less if multiple tube insertions were considered. It was pointed out that the 'collar button' pattern of tube used with these children has a relatively high risk of producing a chronic perforation. It was concluded also that atrophic and calcified scars appeared to be associated with tympanostomy tubes. The issue of whether postero-superior retraction pockets may be caused by tympanostomy tubes was discussed.

It was argued that the migration of tubes from the postero-inferior to the postero-superior position prior to extrusion might, in the presence of continuing negative middle-ear pressure and/or effusion, set the stage for the development of a retraction pocket.

Conclusion

Current knowledge on the epidemiology of OME is inadequate. Very few estimates of the incidence of OME have been reported, and the lack of consistency between those that have raises doubts as to their reliability. Regrettably, the design of the present study precluded the estimation of an incidence rate for the Dunedin population.

Several estimates of the prevalence of OME have been provided from this study. The least useful of these were obtained from the otological histories provided by the parents of the children in the sample. These proved to lack sufficient specificity and reliability to be of value in estimating prevalence. Of much greater use in this regard were the findings of the impedance audiometry and otological examinations conducted at the various phases of the study, with the latter providing a more conservative measure of prevalence than the former.

While the estimates provided by this study of the prevalence of OME in New Zealand children during the early school years are comparable to those reported in northern hemisphere countries, this should not be taken as the final word on the prevalence of the disease. Reliable prevalence estimates are available for very few countries, with those from Denmark tending to dominate the literature. Very few studies have reported prevalence rates for infants. The use of impedance audiometry to determine prevalence has been the dominant method, with very few studies combining methods of identification. Bias in sampling has been identified as a problem in epidemiological studies on OME.

It should be clear from the above comments that considerable research has yet to be done on describing the incidence and prevalence of OME. To be of value, future studies must be designed specifically to yield epidemiological information. Because of the frequently asymptomatic and transient nature of the disease, studies must be prospective, sampling must be representative, identification must involve a combination of impedance audiometry and otoscopy, and observations must commence shortly after birth and be repeated frequently throughout the early childhood years. Furthermore, if geographical differences in the epidemiology of the disease are to be identified then research has to be conducted in many more countries than has been the case up to now.

Finally in this regard, it makes little sense to report prevalence rates in terms of 'ears' rather than 'children', as has frequently been the case in previous studies. If the findings of epidemiological research are to describe accurately the distribution of the disease in a population, and if this information is to be of use to clinicians, health administrators and political decision-makers, then rates per head of population must be reported.

Confirmation has been obtained in this study that the risk of OME is affected significantly by a number of factors including age, sex, season, and some related disorders. The evidence on many other suspected risk factors, however, is not so clear-cut. Furthermore, only rarely do researchers report the relative risk or attributable risk of factors associated with OME. Consequently, while it is widely accepted, for example, that the risk of OME is greater for boys than for girls, neither the degree of increased risk nor the proportion of risk attributable to this factor have been reliably estimated. The need for research designed specifically to produce epidemiological information is just as important in this context as it is in the estimation of incidence and prevalence rates.

The present study has clearly demonstrated the value of longitudinal research in investigating the developmental consequences of OME. Deficits in language development, speech articulation, reading and teacher-reported behaviour problems first identified at 5 years were found to have persisted into the mid-childhood years and were still present at age 11. The difficulties associated with identifying case and comparison groups, which have been a problem in much previous research, are lessened by the longitudinal approach taken here, with the membership of both groups being established at the outset of the study and maintained at subsequent observations. The opportunity for the misclassification of subjects, which exists in retrospective studies, is thereby minimized.

Notwithstanding the necessity for further research on both the epidemiology and developmental consequences of OME, it is evident from the findings of this and other recent studies that there is an urgent need for the detection and management of early onset OME. The work of Jerger *et al.* (1983) and Teele *et al.* (1984) has demonstrated that OME occurring during the first three years of life can significantly delay development in speech, language and social maturity. The present study has shown that delayed speech and language development and behavioural problems associated with OME can persist into the mid-childhood years. From available estimates it is apparent that the prevalence of OME reaches a peak of around 13 per cent by the end of the first year of life and that this level persists throughout the early childhood years. Clearly, a significant proportion of children may be at risk of delays in speech and language development, and have continuing behavioural problems if early onset OME goes undetected and untreated. In contrast to other causes of developmental delays and behavioural problems, therapeutic regimes are readily available for the effective management of OME. The opportunity exists, therefore, for a significant impact to be made on the developmental consequences of OME, through the detection and management of the disease at an early age.

REFERENCES

Asher, M.I., Short, D.P. (1978) 'Child health survey: Ruatoki Family Health Clinic.' (Paper presented to the annual meeting of the Paediatric Society of New Zealand.)

Avery, C.A., Gates, G.A., Prihoda, T.J. (1986) 'Efficacy of acoustic reflectometry in detecting middle ear effusion.' *Annals of Otology Rhinology and Laryngology*, **95**, 472–476.

Bennett, F.C., Ruuska, S.H., Sherman, R. (1980) 'Middle ear function in learning-disabled children.' *Pediatrics*, **66**, 254–260.

Berman, S. (1981) 'Otitis media with effusion. Its relationship to language development, intellectual functioning and academic performance.' *Advances in Behavioural Pediatrics*, **2**, 129–140.

Bess, F.H. (1983) 'Hearing loss associated with middle ear effusion.' *In:* Bluestone, C.D. (Moderator) 'Workshop on effects of otitis media on the child.' *Pediatrics*, **71**, 640–641.

Birch, L., Elbrond, O. (1985) 'Daily impedance audiometric screening of children in a day-care insititution.' *Scandinavian Audiology*, **14**, 5–8.

—— —— (1986) 'Prospective epidemiological study of secretory otitis media in children not attending kindergarten. An incidence study.' *International Journal of Pediatric Otorhinolaryngology*, **11**, 183–90.

—— —— (1987) 'Prospective epidemiological study of common colds and secretory otitis media.' *Clinical Otolaryngology*, **12**, 45–48.

Bishop, D.V.M., Edmundson, A. (1986) 'Is otitis media a major cause of specific developmental language disorders?' *British Journal of Disorders of Communication*, **21**, 321–338.

Black, N.A. (1984) 'Is glue ear a modern phenomenon?—a historical review of the medical literature.' *Clinical Otolaryngology*, **9**, 155–163.

—— (1985) 'The aetiology of glue ear—a case-control study.' *International Journal of Pediatric Otorhinolaryngology*, **9**, 121–133.

Bluestone, C.D. (1980) 'Assessment of eustachian tube function.' *In:* Jerger, J.G., Northern, J.L. (Eds.) *Clinical Impedance Audiometry, 2nd. Edn.* New York: Thieme–Stratton.

—— (1983) 'Effects of otitis media on the child.' *Annals of Otology, Rhinology and Laryngology*, **92** (Suppl. 107), 50.

—— (1984) 'State of the art: Definitions and classifications.' *In:* Lim, D.J., Bluestone, C.D., Klein, J.O., Nelson, J.D. (Eds.) *Recent Advances in Otitis Media with Effusion (Proceedings of the Third International Symposium on Recent Advances in Otitis Media with Effusion).* Philadelphia: Decker.

—— Cantekin, E.I. (1979) 'Design factors in the characterization and identification of otitis media and certain related conditions.' *Annals of Otology, Rhinology and Laryngology*, **88** (Suppl. 60), 13–27.

—— Klein, J.O. (1983) 'Intratemporal complications and sequelae of otitis media.' *In:* Bluestone, C.D., Stool, S.E. (Eds.) *Pediatric Otolaryngology.* Philadelphia: Saunders.

—— Beery, Q.C., Paradise, J.L. (1973) 'Audiometry and tympanometry in relation to middle ear effusions in children.' *Laryngoscope*, **83**, 594–604.

—— Klein, J.O., Paradise, J.L., Eichenwald, H., Bess, F.H., Downs, M.P., Green, M., Berko-Gleason, J., Ventry, I.M., Gray, S.W., McWilliams, B.J., Gates, G.A. (1983) 'Workshop on effects of otitis media on the child.' *Pediatrics*, **71**, 639–652.

Brandes, P.J., Ehinger, D.M. (1981) 'The effects of early middle ear pathology on auditory perception and academic achievement.' *Journal of Speech and Hearing Disorders*, **46**, 250–257.

Brooks, D. N. (1969) 'The use of the electro-acoustic impedance bridge in the assessment of middle ear function.' *International Audiology*, **8**, 563–569.

—— (1979) 'Otitis media and child development: design factors in the identification and assessment of hearing loss.' *Annals of Otology, Rhinology and Laryngology*, **88** (Suppl. 60), 29–47.

—— (1986) 'Otitis media with effusion and academic attainment.' *International Journal of Pediatric Otorhinolaryngology*, **12**, 39–47.

—— (1987) 'Otitis media with effusion: academic attainment and socio-economic background.' *International Journal of Pediatric Otorhinolaryngology*, **13**, 165–170.

Buhrer, K., Wall, L.G., Schuster, L. (1985) 'The acoustic reflectometer as a screening device: a comparison.' *Ear and Hearing*, **6**, 307–314.

Casselbrant, M.L., Okeowo, P.A., Flaherty, R.M., Feldman, R.M., Doyle, W.J., Bluestone, C.D., Rogers, K.D., Hanley, T. (1984) 'Prevalence and incidence of otitis media in a group of preschool children in the United States.' *In:* Lim, D.J., Bluestone, C.D., Klein, J.O., Nelson, J.D. (Eds.), *Recent Advances in Otitis Media with Effusion (Proceedings of the Third International Symposium on Recent Advances in Otitis Media with Effusion).* Philadelphia: Decker.

—— Brostoff, L.M., Cantekin, E.I., Flaherty, M.R., Doyle, W.J., Bluestone, C.D., Fria, T.J. (1985) 'Otitis media with effusion in preschool children.' *Laryngoscope*, **95**, 428–436.
—— —— Ashoff, V.M., Bluestone, C.D. (1986) 'Otitis media in children in the United States.' *In:* Sade, J. (Ed.) *Acute and Secretory Otitis Media (Proceedings of the International Conference on Acute and Secretory Otitis Media—Part 1, Jeruslalem, Israel, 17–22 November, 1985)*. Amsterdam: Kugler.
Clements, C.J., Joseph, J.G. (1981) 'Hearing impairment: causes, effects and prevention.' *New Zealand Health Review*, **1**, 15–19.
Coats, A. (1978) 'Human auditory nerve action potentials and brainstem evoked responses: latency—intensity functions in detection of cochlear and retrocochlear abnormality.' *Archives of Otolaryngology*, **104**, 709–717.
Cook, R.A., Teel, R.W. (1979) 'Negative middle ear pressure and language development.' *Clinical Pediatrics*, **18**, 296–297.
DeSa, D.J. (1973) 'Infection and amniotic aspiration of middle ear in stillbirths and neonatal deaths.' *Archives of Diseases in Childhood*, **48**, 872–880.
—— (1977) 'Polypoidal organization of aspirated amniotic squamous debris (amnion nodosum) in middle-ear cavity of newborn infants.' *Archives of Diseases in Childhood*, **52**, 148–151.
—— (1983) 'Mucosal metaplasia and chronic inflammation in the middle ear of infants receiving intensive care in the neonatal period.' *Archives of Diseases in Childhood*, **58**, 24–28.
Dobie, R.A., Berlin, C.I. (1979) 'Influence of otitis media on hearing and development.' *Annals of Otology, Rhinology and Laryngology*, **88** (Suppl. 60), 48–53.
Downs, M.P. (1982) 'The audiologist and the nonbenign conductive hearing loss of otitis media.' *Seminars in Speech, Language and Hearing*, **3**, 295–304.
—— (1983) 'Audiologist's overview of sequelae of early otitis media.' *In:* Bluestone, C.D. (Moderator) 'Workshop on effects of otitis media on the child.' *Pediatrics*, **71**, 643–644.
Dunn, L. (1965) *The Peabody Picture Vocabulary Test.* Minneapolis: American Guidance Service.
Eaton, D.M., Nowell, H. (1983) 'Reading disability and defects of the middle ear.' *Archives of Diseases in Childhood*, **58**, 1010–1012.
Elley, W.B., Irving, J.C. (1972) 'A socio-economic index for New Zealand based on levels of education and income from the 1966 census.' *New Zealand Journal of Educational Studies*, **7**, 153–167.
—— —— (1976) 'Revised socio-economic index for New Zealand.' *New Zealand Journal of Educational Studies*, **11**, 25–36.
Farmer, R.D.T., Miller, D.L. (1983) *Lecture Notes on Epidemiology and Community Medicine.* Oxford: Blackwell Scientific.
Felding, J.U., Fiellau-Nikolajsen, M., Hojslet, P.E. (1984) 'Impedance as an indicator in irreversible otopathology and hearing loss in nine-year-olds.' *In:* Lim, D.J., Bluestone, C.D., Klein, J.O., Nelson, J.D. (Eds.) *Recent Advances in Otitis Media with Effusion (Proceedings of the Third International Symposium on Recent Advances in Otitis Media with Effusion)*. Philadelphia: Decker.
Fiellau-Nikolajsen, M. (1979) 'Tympanometry in three-year-old children. II: Seasonal influence on tympanometric results in non-selected groups of three-year-old children.' *Scandinavian Audiology*, **8**, 181–185.
—— (1980) 'Tympanometry and middle ear effusion: a cohort study in three-year-old children.' *International Journal of Pediatric Otorhinolaryngology*, **2**, 39–49.
—— (1983*a*) 'Epidemiology of secretory otitis media: a descriptive cohort study.' *Annals of Otology, Rhinology and Laryngology*, **92**, 172–177.
—— (1983*b*) 'Tympanometry and secretory otitis media: observations on diagnosis, epidemiology, treatment, and prevention in prospective cohort studies of three-year-old children. *Acta Oto-Laryngologica*, Suppl. 394.
Fischler, R.S., Todd, W., Feldman, C.M. (1985) 'Otitis media and language performance in a cohort of Apache Indian Children.' *American Journal of Diseases of Childhood*, **139**, 355–360.
Freeman, B.A., Parkins, C. (1979) 'The prevalence of middle ear disease among learning disabled children.' *Clinical Pediatrics*, **18**, 205–212.
Fria, T.J., Cantekin, E.I., Eichler, J.A. (1985) 'Hearing acuity of children with otitis media with effusion.' *Archives of Otolaryngology*, **111**, 10–16.
Friel-Patti, S., Finitzo-Hieber, T., Conti, G., Brown, K.C. (1982) 'Language delay in infants associated with middle ear disease and mild fluctuating hearing impairment.' *Pediatric Infectious Diseases Journal*, **1**, 104–109.
Fundudis, T., Kolvin, I., Garside, R.F. (Eds.). (1979) *Speech Retarded Children: Their Psychological Development.* London: Academic Press.
Gates, G.A., Avery, C., Cooper, J.C., Hearne, E.M., Holt, G.R. (1986) 'Predictive value of tympanometry in middle ear effusion.' *Annals of Otology, Rhinology and Laryngology*, **95**, 46–50.

Giebink, G.S. (1984) 'Epidemiology and natural history of otitis media.' *In:* Lim, D.J., Bluestone, C.D., Klein, J.O., Nelson, J.D. (Eds.) *Recent Advances in Otitis Media with Effusion (Proceedings of the Third International Symposium on Recent Advances in Otitis Media with Effusion).* Philadelphia: Decker.

Golz, A. (1986) 'Reading ability in otitis media children.' *In:* Sade, J. (Ed.) *Acute and Secretory Otitis Media (Proceedings of the International Conference on Acute and Secretory Otitis Media—Part 1, Jerusalem, Israel, 17–22 November, 1985).* Amsterdam: Kugler.

Gottlieb, M.I., Zinkus, P.W., Thompson, A. (1979) 'Chronic middle ear disease and auditory perceptual deficits.' *Clinical Pediatrics*, **18**, 725–732.

Green, D.S. (1978) 'Pure tone air-conduction testing.' *In:* Katz, J. (Ed.) *Handbook of Clinical Audiology.* Baltimore: Williams & Wilkins.

Greville, K.A. (1977) 'The contribution of impedance audiometry to identification of hearing disorders in school children.' (Unpublished M.Sc. thesis, University of Auckland.)

Hall, D.M.B., Hill, P. (1986) 'When does secretory otitis media affect language development?' *Archives of Diseases in Childhood*, **61**, 42–47.

Hamilton, M.A., McKenzie-Pollock, M., Heath, M. (1980) 'Aural health in 227 Northland school and pre-school children.' *New Zealand Medical Journal*, **91**, 59–62.

Haughton, P.M. (1977) 'Validity of tympanometry for middle ear effusions.' *Archives of Otolaryngology*, **103**, 505–513.

Hays, W.L. (1963) *Statistics.* London: Holt, Rinehart & Winston.

Hignett, W. (1983) 'Effects of otitis media on speech, language and behaviour.' *Annals of Otology, Rhinology and Laryngology*, **92** (Suppl. 107), 47–48.

Hoffman-Lawless, K., Keith, R.W., Cotton, R.T. (1981) 'Auditory processing abilities in children with previous middle ear effusion.' *Annals of Otology*, **90**, 543–545.

Holm, V.A., Kunze, L.H. (1969) 'Effect of chronic otitis media on language and speech development.' *Pediatrics*, **43**, 833–839.

Holmquist, J., Al Fadala, S., Gattan, Y. (1987) 'Prevalence of secretory otitis media among school children in Kuwait.' *Journal of Laryngology and Otology*, **101**, 116–119.

Honjo, I., Ushiro, K., Mitoma, T. (1984) 'Endoscopic observation of the eustachian tube in otitis media with effusion.' *In:* Lim, D.J., Bluestone, C.D., Klein, J.O., Nelson, J.D. (Eds.) *Recent Advances in Otitis Media with Effusion (Proceedings of the Third International Symposium on Recent Advances in Otitis Media with Effusion).* Philadelphia: Decker.

Hood, D.A., Elliott, R.B. (1975) 'A comparative study of the health of elite Maori and Caucasian children in Auckland.' *New Zealand Medical Journal*, **81**, 242–243.

Hood, L.J., Faed, J.A., Silva, P.A., Buckfield, P.M. (1978) 'Breast-feeding and some reasons for electing to wean the infant: a report from the Dunedin Multidisciplinary Child Development Study.' *New Zealand Medical Journal*, **88**, 273–276.

Howie, V.M. (1975) 'Natural history of otitis media.' *Annals of Otology, Rhinology and Laryngology*, **84** (Suppl. 19), 67–72.

—— (1979) 'Natural history of otitis media.' *In:* Wiet, R.J., Coulthard, S.W. (Eds). *Proceedings of the Second National Conference on Otitis Media.* Columbus, OH: Ross Laboratories.

—— Ploussard, J.H., Sloyer, J.L. (1976) 'Natural history of otitis media.' *Annals of Otology, Rhinology and Laryngology*, **85** (Suppl. 25), 18–19.

Ingram, T.T.S. (1976) 'Intermittent hearing loss in young children.' *Developmental Medicine and Child Neurology*, **18**, 239–241.

Jaffe, B.F. (1980) 'Amniotic fluid microviscosity and middle ear effusion.' *Pediatrics*, **65**, 362–363.

Jerger, J. (1970) 'Clinical experience with impedance audiometry.' *Archives of Otolaryngology*, **92**, 311–324.

Jerger, S., Jerger, J., Alford, B.R., Abrams, S. (1983) 'Development of speech intelligibility in children with recurrent otitis media.' *Ear and Hearing*, **4**, 138–145.

Jordan, R.E. (1972) 'Epidemiology of otitis media.' *In:* Glorig, A., Gerwin, K.S. (Eds.) *Otitis Media (Proceedings of the National Conference, Gallier Hearing and Speech Centre, Dallas).* Springfield, IL: Charles C. Thomas.

Justin, C., Lawn, L., Silva, P.A. (1983) *The Dunedin Articulation Check (DAC): a Clinical Instrument from the Dunedin Multidisciplinary Health and Development Research Unit.* Dunedin: Otago Speech Therapy Association.

Kaneko, Y., Okitsu, T., Sakuma, M., Shibahara, Y., Yuasa, R., Takasaka, T., Kawamoto, K. (1984) 'Incidence of secretory otitis media after acute inflammation of the middle ear cleft and the upper respiratory tract.' *In:* Lim, D.J., Bluestone, C.D., Klein, J.O., Nelson, J.D. (Eds.) *Recent Advances in Otitis Media with Effusion (Proceedings of the Third International Symposium on Recent Advances in Otitis Media with Effusion).* Philadelphia: Decker.

Kaplan, G.J., Fleshman, J.K., Bender, T.R., Baum, C., Clark, P.S. (1973) 'Long-term effects of otitis media: a ten-year cohort study of Alaskan Eskimo children.' *Pediatrics*, **52**, 577–585.
Kilby, D., Richards, S.H., Hart, G. (1972) 'Grommets and glue ears: two-year results.' *Journal of Laryngology and Otology*, **86**, 881–888.
Kirk, S.A., McCarthy, J.J., Kirk, W.D. (1968) *The Illinois Test of Psycholinguistic Abilities (Revised Edition)*. Urbana, IL: University of Illinois Press.
Klein, J.O. (1979) 'Epidemiology of otitis media.' *In:* Wiet, R.J., Coulthard, S.W. (Eds.) *Proceedings of the Second National Conference on Otitis Media*. Columbus, OH: Ross Laboratories.
—— Henderson, F.W., Keller, M.D. Keller, G., Lanese, R.R., Wiet, R.J. (1980) 'Epidemiology and natural history.' *Annals of Otology, Rhinology and Laryngology*, **89** (Suppl. 69), 4–8.
—— Teele, D.W., Mannos, R., Menyuk, P., Rosner, B.A. (1984) 'Otitis media with effusion during the first three years of life and development of speech and language.' *In:* Lim, D.J., Bluestone, C.D., Klein, J.O., Nelson, J.D. (Eds.) *Recent Advances in Otitis Media with Effusion (Proceedings of the Third International Symposium on Recent Advances in Otitis Media with Effusion)*. Philadelphia: Decker.
Kraemer, M.J., Marshall, S.G., Richardson, M.A. (1984) 'Etiologic factors in the development of chronic middle ear effusions.' *Clinical Review in Allergy*, **2**, 319–328.
Lamothe, A., Boudreault, V., Blanchettė, M., Tetreault, L., Poliquin, J. (1981) 'Serous otitis media: a six week prospective study.' *Journal of Otolaryngology*, **10**, 372–379.
Leiberman, A., Bartal, N. (1986) 'Untreated persistent middle ear effusion.' *Journal of Laryngology and Otology*, **100**, 875–878.
Lewis, N. (1976) 'Otitis media and linguistic competence.' *Archives of Otolaryngology*, **102**, 387–390.
Lilienfeld, A.M., Lilienfeld, D.E. (1980) *Foundations of Epidemiology (2nd. Edn.)*. New York: Oxford University Press.
Lines, D.R. (1977) 'An Auckland high school health survey.' *Australia and New Zealand Journal of Medicine*, **7**, 143–147.
Lous, J. (1986) 'Linguistic and cognitive sequelae to secretory otitis media in children.' *Scandinavian Audiology*, **26** (Suppl.), 71–75.
—— Fiellau-Nikolajsen, M. (1981) 'Epidemiology of middle ear effusion and tubal dysfunction. A one-year prospective study comprising monthly tympanometry in 387 non-selected 7 year-old children.' *International Journal of Pediatric Otorhinolaryngology*, **3**, 303–317.
—— —— (1984a) 'A 5-year prospective case-control study of the influence of early otitis media with effusion on reading achievement.' *International Journal of Pediatric Otorhinolaryngology*, **8**, 19–30.
—— —— (1984b) 'Influence of early otitis media with effusion on reading achievement: a five-year prospective case-control study.' *In:* Lim, D.J., Bluestone, C.D., Klein, J.O., Nelson, J.D. (Eds.) *Recent Advances in Otitis Media with Effusion (Proceedings of the Third International Symposium on Recent Advances in Otitis Media with Effusion)*. Philadelphia: Decker.
McDermott, J.C. (1983) 'Physical and behavioural aspects of middle ear disease in school children.' *Journal of School Health*, **53**, 463–466.
McGee, R.O., Silva, P.A. (1982) *A Thousand New Zealand Children: Their Health and Development from Birth to Seven (Special Report Series, No. 8)*. Auckland: Medical Research Council of New Zealand.
—— —— Williams, S.M. (1983) 'Parents' and teachers' perception of behaviour problems in seven year old children.' *Exceptional Child*, **30**, 151–161.
—— —— —— (1984) 'Perinatal, neurological, environmental and developmental characteristics of seven-year-old children with stable behaviour problems.' *Journal of Child Psychology and Psychiatry*, **25**, 573–586.
Marchant, C.D., McMillan, P.M., Shurin, P.A., Johnson, C.E., Turczyk, V.A., Feinstein, J.C., Panek, D.M. (1986) 'Objective diagnosis of otitis media in early infancy by tympanometry and ipsilateral acoustic reflex thresholds.' *Journal of Pediatrics*, **109**, 590–595.
Marshall, S.G., Furukawa, C.T., Pierson, W.E., Shapiro, G.G., Bierman, C.W. (1984) 'Prevalence of middle ear dysfunction and otitis media with effusion in atopic children.' *In:* Lim, D.J., Bluestone, C.D., Klein, J.O., Nelson, J.D. (Eds.) *Recent Advances in Otitis Media with Effusion (Proceedings of the Third International Symposium on Recent Advances in Otitis Media with Effusion)*. Philadelphia: Decker.
Martin, F. (1981) *Introduction to Audiology, 2nd. Edn*. Englewood Cliffs, NJ: Prentice Hall.
Masters, L., Marsh, G.E. (1978) 'Middle ear pathology as a factor in learning disabilities.' *Journal of Learning Disabilities*, **11**, 54–57.
Mawson, S.R. (1976) 'Middle ear effusions: definitions.' *Annals of Otology, Rhinology and Laryngology*, **85** (Suppl. 25), 12–14.
Maynard, E.J., Keith, W.J. (1981) *Hearing Screening Amongst New School Entrants*. South Auckland:

South Auckland District Health Office (unpublished report).
Menyuk, P. (1979) 'Design factors in the assessment of language development in children with otitis media.' *Annals of Otology, Rhinology and Laryngology*, **88** (Suppl. 60), 78–87.
—— (1980) 'Effects of persistent otitis media on language development.' *Annals of Otology, Rhinology and Laryngology*, **89** (Suppl. 68), 257–263.
Mills, R.P., Uttley, A.H.C., McIntyre, M.F., Brain, C.E. (1986) 'The role of acute suppurative otitis media in the pathogenesis of chronic middle ear effusions.' *In:* Sade, J. (Ed.) *Acute and Secretory Otitis Media (Proceedings of the International Conference on Acute and Secretory Otitis Media—Part 1, Jerusalem, Israel, 17–22 November, 1985)*. Amsterdam: Kugler.
Mustain, W.D. (1979) 'Linguistic and educational implications of recurrent otitis media.' *Ear, Nose and Throat Journal*, **58**, 218–222.
Needleman, H. (1977) 'Effects of hearing loss from early recurrent otitis media on speech and language development.' *In:* Jaffe, B. (Ed.) *Hearing Loss in Children*. Baltimore: University Park Press.
New Zealand Board of Health Committee on Hearing (1984) *The Hearing Report: Findings and Initial Recommendations of the Board of Health Committee on Hearing*. Wellington: New Zealand Board of Health.
Northern, J.L., Downs, M.P. (1978) *Hearing in Children, 2nd. Edn.* Baltimore: Williams & Wilkins.
—— Grimes, A.M. (1978) 'Introduction to acoustic impedance.' *In:* Katz, J. (Ed.) *Handbook of Clinical Audiology*. Baltimore: Williams & Wilkins.
Okeowo, P.A. (1985) 'Observations on the incidence of secretory otitis media in Nigerian children.' *Journal of Tropical Pediatrics*, **31**, 295–298.
Orchik, D.J., Morff, R., Dunn, J.W. (1978) 'Impedance audiometry in serous otitis media.' *Archives of Otolaryngology*, **104**, 409–412.
Oyiborhoro, J.M.A., Olaniyan, S.O., Newman, C.W., Balakrishnan, S.L. (1987) 'Efficacy of acoustic otoscope in detecting middle ear effusion in children.' *Laryngoscope*, **97**, 495–498.
Paden, E.P., Novak, M.A., Beiter, A.L. (1987) 'Predictors of phonologic inadequacy in young children prone to otitis media.' *Journal of Speech and Hearing Disorders*, **52**, 232–242.
Paparella, M.M. (1976) 'Middle ear effusions: definitions and terminology.' *Annals of Otology, Rhinology and Laryngology*, **85** (Suppl. 25), 8–11.
—— Bluestone, C.D., Arnold, W., et al. (1985) 'Definition and classification.' *Annals of Otology, Rhinology and Laryngology*, **94** (Suppl. 116), 8–9.
Paradise, J.L. (1976) 'Pediatrician's view of middle ear effusions: more questions than answers.' *Annals of Otology, Rhinology and Laryngology*, **85** (Suppl. 25), 20–24.
—— (1980) 'Otitis media in infants and children.' *Pediatrics*, **65**, 917–943.
—— (1981) 'Otitis media during early life: how hazardous to development? A critical review of the evidence.' *Pediatrics*, **68**, 869–873.
—— (1983) 'Long-term effects of short-term hearing loss—menace or myth?' *Pediatrics*, **71**, 647–648.
—— Rodgers, K.D. (1980) 'Ubiquitous otitis media: a child health problem of uncertain dimensions.' *American Journal of Public Health*, **70**, 577–578.
—— Smith C.G. (1979) 'Impedance screening for preschool children.' *Annals of Otology*, **88**, 56–65.
Poulsen, G., Tos, M. (1978) 'Screening tympanometry in newborn infants and during the first six months of life.' *Scandinavian Audiology*, **7**, 159–166.
Rach, G.H., Zielhuis, G.A., van den Broek, P. (1986) 'The prevalence of otitis media with effusion in two-year old children in the Netherlands.' *In:* Sade, J. (Ed.) *Acute and Secretory Otitis Media (Proceedings of the International Conference on Acute and Secretory Otitis Media—Part 1, Jerusalem, Israel, 17–22 November, 1985)*. Amsterdam: Kugler.
Rapin, I. (1979) 'Conductive hearing loss effects on children's language and scholastic skills: a review of the literature.' *Annals of Otology, Rhinology and Laryngology*, **88** (Suppl. 60), 3–11.
Reichman, J., Healey, W.C. (1983) 'Learning disabilities and conductive hearing loss involving otitis media.' *Journal of Learning Disabilities*, **16**, 272–278.
Renvall, U., Aniansson, G., Liden, G. (1982) 'Spontaneous improvement in ears with middle ear disease.' *International Journal of Pediatric Otorhinolaryngology*, **4**, 245–250.
—— Jarlstedt, J., Holmquist, J. (1980) 'Identification of middle ear disease.' *Acta Otolaryngologica*, **90**, 283–289.
Reves, R., Budgett, R., Miller, D., Wadsworth, J., Haines, A. (1985) 'Study of middle ear disease using tympanometry in general practice.' *British Medical Journal*, **290**, 1953–1956.
Reynell, J. (1969) *Reynell Developmental Language Scales*. London: National Foundation for Educational Research.
Roberts, J.E., Sanyal, M.A., Burchinal, M.R., Collier, A.M., Ramey, C.T., Henderson, F.W. (1986) 'Otitis media in early childhood and its relationship to later verbal and academic performance.' *Pediatrics*, **78**, 423–430.

Rockley, T.J., Rhys Evans, P.H. (1986) 'Secretory otitis media—evidence for an inherited aetiology.' *Journal of Laryngology and Otology*, **100**, 389–393.
Ruben, R.J., Hanson, D.G. (1979) 'Summary of discussion and recommendations made during the workshop on otitis media and development.' *Annals of Otology, Rhinology and Laryngology*, **88** (Suppl. 60), 107–111.
Rutter, M., Tizard, J., Whitmore, K. (1970) *Education, Health and Behaviour.* London: Longman.
Sak, R.J., Ruben, R.J. (1981) 'Recurrent middle ear effusion in childhood: implications of temporary auditory deprivation for language and learning.' *Annals of Otology*, **90**, 546–551.
Scheffe, H. (1953) 'A method for judging all contrasts in an analysis of variance.' *Biometrika*, **40**, 87–104.
Schwartz, D.M., Schwartz, R.H. (1987) 'Validity of acoustic reflectometry in detecting middle ear effusion.' *Pediatrics*, **79**, 739–742.
Scottish Council for Research in Education (1976) *The Burt Word Reading Test (1974 Revision).* London: Hodder & Stoughton.
Sears, M., Jones, D.T., Holdaway, M.D., Hewitt, C.J., Flannery, E.M., Herbison, G.P., Silva, P.A. (1986) 'Prevalence of bronchial reactivity to inhaled methacholine in New Zealand children.' *Thorax*, **41**, 283–289.
Senturia, B.H. (1976) 'Classification of middle ear effusions.' *Annals of Otology, Rhinology and Laryngology*, **85** (Suppl. 25), 15–17.
—— Paparella, M.M., Lowery, H.W., *et al.* (1980) 'Definition and classification.' *In:* Lim, D.J. (Ed.) 'Report of research conference: recent advances in otitis media with effusion.' *Annals of Otology, Rhinology and Laryngology*, **89** (Suppl. 69), 4–8.
Silva, P.A. (1980) *The Dunedin Articulation Screening Scale (DASS).* Dunedin: Otago Speech Therapy Association.
—— Fergusson, D.M. (1976) 'Socio-economic status, maternal characteristics, child experience and intelligence in preschool children.' *New Zealand Journal of Educational Studies*, **11**, 180–188.
—— Kirkland, C., Simpson, A., Stewart, I.A., Williams, S.M. (1982) 'Some developmental and behavioural characteristics associated with bilateral otitis media with effusion.' *Journal of Learning Disabilities*, **15**, 417–421.
—— McGee, R., Williams, S. (1981) *From Birth to Seven: Child Development in Dunedin. A Multidisciplinary Study. (Report to the Medical Research Council of New Zealand, The National Children's Health Research Foundation, The Department of Education and the Department of Health.)* (Unpublished report, available from University of Otago Medical Library.)
—— —— —— (1983) 'Developmental language delay from three to seven years and its significance for low intelligence and reading difficulties at age seven.' *Developmental Medicine and Child Neurology*, **25**, 783–793.
—— Spears, G., Williams, S. (1984) *A Description of the Dunedin Multidisciplinary Child Development Study Data Set: Phases I to XI.* Dunedin: Dunedin Multidisciplinary Health and Development Research Unit.
SPSS Incorporated (1983) *SPSS-X Users Guide.* New York: McGraw–Hill.
Stangerup, S.-E., Tos, M. (1985) 'The etiologic role of acute suppurative otitis media in chronic secretory otitis.' *American Journal of Otology*, **6**, 126–131.
Stanhope, J.M., Aitchison, W.R., Swindells, J.C., Frankish, J.D. (1978) 'Ear disease in rural New Zealand school children.' *New Zealand Medical Journal*, **88**, 5–11.
Stewart, I.A. (1980) 'Secretory otitis media and unsuspected hearing loss in children.' *Patient Management*, **9** (5), 35–43.
—— (1981) 'Otological problems.' *In:* Silva, P.A., McGee, R., Williams, S. (Eds.) *From Birth to Seven.* (Unpublished research report available from the University of Otago Medical Library.)
—— Jenkin, L., Kirkland, C., Silva, P., Simpson, A. (1983) 'A preliminary evaluation of the use of an automatic impedance tympanometer in the diagnosis of otitis media with effusion in children: a report from The Dunedin Multidisciplinary Health and Development Research Unit.' *New Zealand Medical Journal*, **96**, 252–255.
—— Silva, P.A., Said, S., Takazawa, A., Webster, G., White, P., Williams, S.M. (1989) 'Attic and posterior marginal retractions in a random sample of 794 children.' *In:* Tos, M. *et al.* (Eds.) *Proceedings of the Third International Conference on Cholesteatoma and Mastoid Surgery.* Amsterdam: Kugler & Ghedini. *(In press.)*
Stickler, G.B. (1984) 'The attack on the tympanic membrane.' *Pediatrics*, **74**, 291–292.
Sunderman, J., Dyer, H. (1984) 'Chronic ear disease in Australian Aborigines.' *Medical Journal of Australia*, **140**, 708–711.
Teele, D.W., Teele, J. (1984) 'Detection of middle ear effusion by acoustic reflectometry.' *In:* Lim, D.J., Bluestone, C.D., Klein, J.O., Nelson, J.D. (Eds.) *Recent Advances in Otitis Media with*

Effusion (Proceedings of the Third International Symposium on Recent Advances in Otitis Media with Effusion). Philadelphia: Decker.

—— Klein, J.O., Rosner, B., and the Greater Boston Otitis Media Study Group (1981) 'Effects of middle ear effusion on development of speech and language.' *Pediatric Research*, **15**, 623. (Abstract no. 1082.)

—— —— —— and the Greater Boston Otitis Media Study Group (1984) 'Otitis media with effusion during the first three years of life and development of speech and language.' *Pediatrics*, **74**, 282–287.

Terman, L.M., Merrill, M.A. (1960) *Stanford–Binet Intelligence Scale (Manual for the Third Revision, Form L-M)*. Boston: Houghton Mifflin.

Thompson, J., Wright, P.F., Greene, J.W., Andrews, C.S., Vaughn, W.K., Sitton, A., McConnell, K.B., Sell, S.H., Bess, F.H. (1984) 'Natural history of acute and serous otitis media during the first two years of life.' *In:* Lim, D.J., Bluestone, C.D., Klein, J.O., Nelson, J.D. (Eds.) *Recent Advances in Otitis Media with Effusion (Proceedings of the Third International Symposium on Recent Advances in Otitis Media with Effusion)*. Philadelphia: Decker.

Tonkin, S.L. (1977) 'Tokelau Island children's study: common diseases.' *In:* Stanhope, J. (Ed.) *Migration and Health in New Zealand and the Pacific*. Wellington: Wellington Hospital Epidemiology Unit.

Tos, M. (1980) 'Spontaneous improvement of secretory otitis and impedance screening.' *Archives of Otolaryngology*, **106**, 345–349.

—— (1983) 'Epidemiology and spontaneous improvement of secretory otitis.' *Acta Oto-Rhino-Laryngologica Belgica*, **37**, 31–43.

—— Poulsen, G. (1979) 'Tympanometry in 2-year-old children: seasonal influence on frequency of secretory otitis and tubal function.' *ORL: Journal of Oto-Rhino-Laryngology and its Related Specialities*, **41**, 1–10.

—— —— (1980) 'Attic retractions following secretory otitis.' *Acta Otolaryngologica*, **89**, 479–486.

—— Bonding, P., Poulsen, G. (1983*a*) 'Tympanosclerosis of the drum in secretory otitis after insertion of grommets.' *Journal of Laryngology and Otology*, **97**, 489–496.

—— Holm-Jensen, S., Stangerup, S.E., Sorensen, C.H. (1983*b*) 'Changes in point prevalence of secretory otitis in preschool children.' *ORL: Journal of Oto-Rhino-Laryngology and its Related Specialities*, **45**, 226–234.

—— Poulsen, G., Borch, J. (1978) 'Tympanometry in two year old children.' *ORL: Journal of Oto-Rhino-Laryngology and its Related Specialities*, **40**, 77–85.

—— —— —— (1979*a*) 'Etiologic factors in secretory otitis.' *Archives of Otolaryngology*, **105**, 582–588.

—— —— Hancke, A.B. (1979b) 'Screening tympanometry during the first year of life.' *Acta Otolaryngologica*, **88**, 388–394.

—— Stangerup, S., Andreassen, U.K., Hvid, G., Thomsen, J., Holm-Jensen, S. (1984) 'Natural history of secretory otitis media.' *In:* Lim, D.J., Bluestone, C.D., Klein, J.O., Nelson, J.D. (Eds.) *Recent Advances in Otitis Media with Effusion (Proceedings of the Third International Symposium on Recent Advances in Otitis Media with Effusion)*. Philadelphia: Decker.

Van Cauwenberge, P.B. (1986) 'Otitis media in relation to other upper respiratory tract infections.' *In:* Sade, J. (Ed.) *Acute and Secretory Otitis Media (Proceedings of the International Conference on Acute and Secretory Otitis Media—Part 1, Jerusalem, Israel, 17–22 November, 1985)*. Amsterdam: Kugler.

—— Kluyskens, P.M. (1984) 'Some predisposing factors in otitis media with effusion.' *In:* Lim, D.J., Bluestone, C.D., Klein, J.O., Nelson, J.D. (Eds.) *Recent Advances in Otitis Media with Effusion (Proceedings of the Third International Symposium on Recent Advances in Otitis Media with Effusion)*. Philadelphia: Decker.

—— Declercq, G., Kluyskens, P.M. (1986*a*) 'The relationship between acute and secretory otitis media.' *In:* Sade, J. (Ed.) *Acute and Secretory Otitis Media (Proceedings of the International Conference on Acute and Secretory Otitis Media—Part 1, Jerusalem, Israel, 17–22 November, 1985)*. Amsterdam: Kugler.

—— Derycke, A., Kluyskens, P.M. (1986*b*) 'The influence of secretory and acute otitis media on speech and language development and psycho-social behaviour.' *In:* Sade, J. (Ed.) *Acute and Secretory Otitis Media (Proceedings of the International Conference on Acute and Secretory Otitis Media—Part 1, Jerusalem, Israel, 17–22 November, 1985)*. Amsterdam: Kugler.

—— Van Cauwenberge, K., Kluyskens, P. (1985) 'The influence of otitis media with effusion on speech and language development and psycho-intellectual behaviour of the preschool child—results of a cross-sectional study in 1,512 children.' *Auris Nasus Larynx*, **12** (Suppl. 1), S228–S230.

Ventry, I.M. (1980) 'Effects of conductive hearing loss: fact or fiction?' *Journal of Speech and Hearing Disorders*, **45**, 143–156.

—— (1983) 'Research design issues in studies of effects of middle ear effusion.' *In:* Bluestone, C.D.

(Moderator) 'Workshop on effects of otitis media on the child.' *Pediatrics,* **71**, 644.
Visscher, W., Mandel, J.S., Batalden, P.B., Russ, J.M., Giebink, G.S. (1984) 'A case-control study exploring possible risk factors for childhood otitis media.' *In:* Lim, D.J., Bluestone, C.D., Klein, J.O., Nelson, J.D. (Eds.) *Recent Advances in Otitis Media with Effusion (Proceedings of the Third International Symposium on Recent Advances in Otitis Media with Effusion).* Philadelphia: Decker.
Wechsler, D. (1974) *The Wechsler Intelligence Scale for Children—Revised.* New York: Psychological Corporation.
Wright, P.F., McConnell, K.B., Thompson, J.M., Vaughn, W.K., Sell, S.H. (1985) 'A longitudinal study of the detection of otitis media in the first two years of life.' *International Journal of Pediatric Otorhinolaryngology*, **10**, 245–252.
Zinkus, P.W. (1982) 'Psychoeducational sequelae of chronic otitis media.' *Seminars in Speech, Language and Hearing*, **3**, 305–312.
—— Gottlieb, M.I. (1980) 'Patterns of perceptual and academic deficits related to early chronic otitis media.' *Pediatrics*, **66**, 246–253.
—— —— Schapiro, M. (1978) 'Developmental and psychoeducational sequelae of chronic otitis media.' *American Journal of Diseases of Children*, **132**, 1100–1104.

INDEX